CONTROLLING

IBS

THE DRUG-FREE WAY

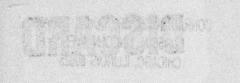

CONTROLLING
IBS
THE DRUG-FREE WAY

A 10-STEP PLAN FOR SYMPTOM RELIEF

DR. JEFFREY M. LACKNER

Director, Behavioral Medicine Clinic
University at Buffalo School of Medicine, SUNY

STEWART, TABORI & CHANG
NEW YORK

Published in 2007 by Stewart, Tabori & Chang
An imprint of Harry N. Abrams, Inc.

The ideas, procedures, and suggestions contained in this book are not intended
as a substitute for consultation with a health-care professional. Each individual's
health concerns should be evaluated by a qualified professional.

Library of Congress Cataloging-in-Publication Data
Lackner, Jeffrey M.
  Controlling IBS the drug-free way : a 10-step plan for symptom relief /
Jeffrey M. Lackner.
      p. cm.
   ISBN 978-1-58479-575-9
  1. Irritable colon–Popular works. 2. Irritable colon–Treatment–Popular
works. 3. Irritable colon–Alternative treatment–Popular works. 4.
Self-care, Health. I. Title.

RC862.I77L3358 2007
616.3'42–dc22

                                    2007013424

EDITOR Julie Stillman
COVER, BOOK DESIGN, AND COMPOSITION by Michelle Farinella Design
PRODUCTION MANAGER Tina Cameron

The text of this book was composed in Sabon.
Printed and bound in the United States of America
10 9 8 7 6 5 4 3 2 1

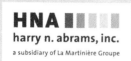

HNA
harry n. abrams, inc.
a subsidiary of La Martinière Groupe

115 West 18th Street
New York, NY 10011
www.hnabooks.com

For Ann Marie, with love

CONTENTS

Officially, from a physician's viewpoint irritable bowel syndrome (IBS) is a common so-called "functional" disorder characterized by chronic abdominal pain and discomfort associated with changes in bowel habits. Other than ruling out "something serious" by blood and stool tests, or by referring the patient to a gastroenterologist for a colonoscopy, the busy physician has little to offer in terms of effective medications or even time to listen, and generally has little interest to follow a patient, once a diagnosis of IBS is established. Well-intentioned phone calls and routine follow-up visits on the part of the frustrated patient are treated by the medical community as "illness behaviors," "excessive health-care seeking," or as a neurotic preoccupation with bowel habits.

But from the patient's standpoint, the perspective couldn't be more different. Many patients suffer from their GI symptoms to a degree that compromises their ability to lead normal lives, and they are frustrated by the medical system's inability to find a cause for, or treat their symptoms effectively. Often after seeking medical help, many patients leave the doctor's office without any plausible explanation for what causes their symptoms and without specific treatment recommendations. If it weren't for some highly effective patient support organizations, such as the International Foundation for Functional GI Disorders (IFFGD), many patients would be forced to suffer silently with their condition. To make matters worse, despite a sustained and laudable effort by the pharmaceutical industry during the past 15 years, very few new medications have been developed for IBS, and those that turned out to be helpful were either withdrawn or severely restricted in response to the FDA's concern about safety. This has further heightened the feelings of helplessness and frustration for those who suffer from IBS.

Here is where Dr. Lackner's book comes in. Among the growing number of IBS self-help books and websites, it is rare to find such an authoritative, scientifically up-to-date, and easily understandable book that ultimately empowers the patient. From the initial overview of the science behind IBS, the book guides readers through a 10-step program that provides them with practical skills to gain control of their IBS symptoms. This is a source of information that many patients wish they had access to 10 years ago! What makes this book even stronger is the fact that Dr. Lackner has already demonstrated in high-quality clinical trials that a behavioral self- management approach really works, even for the most severe forms of IBS.

Some skeptical patients may glance over the table of contents and come to the premature conclusion that this book is all about "psychological stuff" that is not going to work for them, since they don't have a psychological problem but suffer from a "real" disease whose symptoms are neither "all in your head" nor call for a psychiatrist. However, there are several strong arguments against such skepticism. First, the book aims to put patients back in the driver's seat— rather than being a victim of their symptoms, they first learn to understand what causes them, how to identify symptom triggers, and how to gain control over them. Second, the book aims to empower patients to become experts who understand all their symptoms, the underlying mechanisms, and the tools needed to reduce symptoms. Third, recent scientific breakthroughs exploring just how the brain and gut interact suggest that the skills featured in this book may not only relieve symptoms, but may do so by "rewiring" the brain circuitry underlying IBS symptoms.

I wouldn't be surprised if the majority of IBS patients reading this book will wonder why nobody has given them this information before, and will be impressed by their ability to learn ways to train the mind to control this chronic, painful, and often debilitating disorder. Those who struggle with IBS will find this book a valuable resource, as will the health-care professionals who treat them.

Emeran A. Mayer, M.D.
Professor and Director
Center for Neurovisceral Sciences & Women's Health
Division of Digestive Diseases
David Geffen School of Medicine at UCLA

ACKNOWLEDGMENTS

THERE ARE SEVERAL GROUPS OF PEOPLE to whom I wish to express my gratitude. This book is an extension of over 20 years of IBS research that was largely conducted by Edward Blanchard and his students at the University at Albany, SUNY. Ed's generosity, kindness, and guidance are greatly appreciated. Four individuals whose research efforts shape the structure, spirit, and content of this book are Terry Wilson, Ken Holroyd, David Barlow, and Tom Borkovec.

I am grateful for the financial support of the National Institute of Diabetes, Digestive and Kidney Diseases (NIDDK) of the National Institutes of Health. Special thanks are due Patricia Robuck, Director of NIDDK's Clinical Trials Program, for challenging me to help develop innovative, clinically meaningful and practical behavioral self-management treatments, test them under scientifically rigorous conditions, and disseminate them in the "real world" where the vast majority of IBS patients struggle without satisfactory relief from symptoms.

I am fortunate to have had wonderful colleagues/friends within the University at Buffalo's Division of Gastroenterology (Department of Medicine) and its Behavioral Medicine Clinic. I would particularly like to mention Susan Krasner, Rebecca Firth, Leonard Katz, Michael Sitrin, Gregory Gudleski, Catherine Powell, Praveen Sampath, Katy Dorsheimer, Caroline Tidwell, Deborah Hembrook, and Ann Marie Carosella. Without them, this book would not exist.

Thanks to Emeran Mayer and Bruce Naliboff for their support.

I am grateful to the many patients who have participated in our clinical research programs at UB. Their honesty, hard work, and willingness to share their experiences with IBS gives the book its heart, soul, and guts. I gratefully acknowledge the help of Laurie Keefer and Irwin Rosenberg for their careful reviews of portions of the book for scientific accuracy.

To Rachel and Benjamin, thank you for quieting down long (and often) enough for daddy to get through this—I will make it up to you both.

Leslie Stoker at Stewart, Tabori & Chang deserves my appreciation for seeing value in converting the clinical materials of our research protocol into a trade book accessible to a wider audience. I thank Carol Turkington, whose courage in the face of adversity is as much admired as the contributions she made to multiple drafts of this book. Finally, I thank my editor, Julie Stillman, for her constructive criticisms, patience, attention to detail, poise, and shrewd hockey sense.

PART ONE

WHAT IS IBS?

As many as 40 million Americans suffer from irritable bowel syndrome. For the great majority, the symptoms are manageable, infrequent, and not disabling. But 10 million people find symptoms a nearly constant source of physical and mental strain that doesn't get better with medication or dietary changes. If you are one of these people, this book was written for you. It is designed to help you learn how to control IBS symptoms. The first step in taking an active role in managing IBS is learning as much about it as you can. The first chapter will help you understand IBS: what it is and isn't, what causes it, how it is diagnosed, who suffers with it, and how it is different from other gastrointestinal problems with similar symptoms. This chapter separates fact from fiction to give you the most current, scientifically accurate information about IBS. The second chapter gives you an overview of the 10-step plan developed and tested at the State University of New York, which is the core of this book. You will learn that regardless of how IBS symptoms begin, they are often fueled by a vicious cycle of physical, behavioral, and environmental factors that disrupt the neural connections linking the brain and gut. Our goal is to give you a set of practical tools that reverse this cycle, thereby decreasing symptoms and helping you reclaim your life.

IBS: WHAT'S IT ALL ABOUT?

*Jane was 28 when she was diagnosed with irritable bowel syndrome (IBS),
although she'd been suffering with symptoms since she was 15. "It started
off with the occasional stomach cramp and has gotten worse over the past
five years. My bowels are totally out of whack. I cycle from bad diarrhea
to constipation several times a year, but my symptoms never really let up,"
she says. The worst part about having IBS, she believes, is the toll it takes
on her social life. "I can't commit to anything too far in advance. IBS
makes you feel like a dog leashed to a pole. Inevitably, as I'm gearing up for
a special event, I'm stuck in the bathroom. When I finally arrive, I'm on the
lookout for the closest restroom and I don't dare veer too far away. I
never know when I might have another flare-up. My stomach has taken
over my life. It affects what I do, the way I feel, how I think about things.
Sometimes I just want to scream 'Enough already!' Don't I deserve a break
from this?"*

Unfortunately, Jane's symptoms aren't unique. One out of every five adult
Americans—nearly 40 million people—share Jane's symptoms of irritable
bowel syndrome (IBS). Whether it occurs on the job, on vacation, or
during recreation, IBS affects nearly every aspect of your life.

In fact, IBS is the most common illness diagnosed by gastroenterologists, and one of the most common disorders seen by primary care
physicians, even though only a small group of people with symptoms
actually seek medical help. In fact, only one out of every four people with
IBS symptoms *ever* consults a physician.

Why so many people are reluctant to seek help isn't entirely clear. Some
are simply too embarrassed to ask for help; others aren't sure where to go
for treatment or what kind of treatment really works. Still others don't
realize their symptoms are part of a treatable condition. Others have
lost confidence in traditional medical options and have turned to unproven
home remedies, herbal products, and over-the-counter medicines in a
desperate search for relief.

Far too many patients who *have* consulted a doctor are told that there's nothing wrong, and "you'll just have to learn to live with it," and so they resign themselves to a life of pain and suffering. Unfortunately, they don't know that with proper treatment, they can feel better and actually get their lives back to normal.

WHAT ARE THE SYMPTOMS OF IBS?

If you struggle with IBS, you're probably all too aware of the impact it can have on your life. IBS isn't just an upset stomach or episode of diarrhea or constipation that crops up every now and then. It's a real medical condition. If you have IBS, you'll experience abdominal pain or discomfort along with irregular bowel habits such as chronic diarrhea, constipation, or both. However, the nature of the primary bowel problem often differs from one person to the next.

For many people, IBS symptoms are nothing more than an occasional nuisance. For others, symptoms are so severe that they are a debilitating source of physical and emotional strain that disrupts relationships with family and friends, diminishes productivity, leads to frequent absences from work and school, taxes financial resources, and even affects mood and self-confidence. In fact, more than 25 percent of people with IBS find that symptoms restrict their ability to lead a normal life on at least a weekly basis. Indeed, research has found that IBS patients report a lower quality of life than those diagnosed with chronic illnesses such as diabetes, arthritis, and stroke.

Typically, people with IBS complain of changes in bowel habits, including diarrhea, constipation, or both. *Diarrhea* refers to an increase in the frequency of bowel movements or a loose stool. People who have diarrhea describe their stool as loose, watery, and frequent (more than three times in one day.) Although changes in the frequency of bowel movements and looseness of stool don't necessarily go hand in hand, these changes usually occur together. Diarrhea usually occurs during the day and is often preceded by a strong sense of urgency to move the bowels.

There is no single definition of constipation but it is generally described as infrequent defecation. If you're constipated, your stool is usually hard, dry, small, and difficult to pass. Some people who are constipated find it painful to have a bowel movement or feel they haven't evacuated their bowels fully, even when the rectum is truly empty. This can lead to straining during a bowel movement or spending a lot of time sitting on the toilet.

About a third of people with IBS have a predominant component of constipation, called *constipation-predominant IBS*. Another third struggle with diarrhea, and fall into a group called *diarrhea-predominant IBS*. The final third alternate between bouts of constipation and diarrhea. Some patients swing from constipation-predominant IBS to diarrhea-predominant IBS and back again. Many people's symptoms do not fall neatly into any one category, and there is much overlap between categories. The fluctuating complexion of bowel problems has made it hard to develop a single drug to tackle all the symptoms of IBS over time, and emphasizes the importance of doing everything you can to take control of your symptoms.

Of course, having bowel movements three times a day or three times a week doesn't necessarily mean you have a problem with diarrhea, constipation, or IBS. If an IBS diagnosis were based simply on whether you had a bowel movement fewer than three times a week or more than three times a day, 95 percent of Americans would be diagnosed with IBS! Because bowel movements are so variable and because there's no ironclad rule about exactly how many bowel movements constitute diarrhea or constipation, experts believe it's more helpful to focus on the consistency of the stool, the effort required to pass a bowel movement, and changes in the frequency of bowel movements from your usual pattern.

In addition to changes in bowel habits, IBS is characterized by abdominal discomfort or pain that comes and goes. In fact, abdominal discomfort is a symptom common to all types of IBS. Not only is pain uncomfortable and potentially disabling, but it is usually the IBS symptom that triggers a patient's decision to seek medical attention. Many IBS patients describe the pain as dull, crampy, or sharp, typically located in the lower left part of the abdomen. However, what the pain feels like, how severe it is, and where it's located differ from person to person. Some patients find that pain occurs anywhere in the abdominal area; others find that the pain is specific to one site. Some IBS patients find that pain initially begins in one spot and then "spreads" across a larger part of the abdomen. Other symptoms associated with IBS may include bloating, gas, mucus in the stool, or a sense of urgency (having to go to the bathroom immediately). Some people feel an urgent need to head to the toilet, often several times after waking in the morning—this can often occur after breakfast.

IBS can take a toll on your body, your feelings, your thoughts, and your behavior. It can cloud the way you think about the world, make you feel miserable, and create an invisible wall between you and your loved ones. But IBS isn't a mental illness, and the symptoms aren't emotional or "all in your head." Bowel symptoms aren't a sign of personal weakness or a condition that can be willed or wished away. *It's not your fault you have IBS.*

IBS is a real medical problem, even though nothing abnormal shows up on X-rays or blood tests. In IBS, the digestive tract isn't working the way it should. The muscles may contract too forcefully or quickly at some times, too slowly or weakly at other times. The symptoms that accompany IBS can be so unpleasant that you may wonder whether you have cancer or a life-threatening or progressive medical illness that will get worse if you don't treat it. This is why some people often seek medical attention when their symptoms flare up, and undergo extensive medical tests to rule out other conditions that mimic symptoms of IBS.

Of course, patients aren't the only ones confused by IBS symptoms.

According to a study published in the medical journal *Gastroenterology*, people with IBS symptoms are at higher risk for undergoing needless surgeries—gall bladder removals, hysterectomies, appendectomies— because their doctors are also confused by what GI symptoms mean.

Bowel problems are not the only medical problem afflicting people with IBS symptoms. IBS patients are twice as likely to be diagnosed with nongastrointestinal medical problems as non-IBS patients. These include headache, low back pain, arthritis, muscle pain, skin rash, poor sleep, chronic fatigue syndrome, and sexual difficulties. These medical problems can be a source of emotional, physical, and financial strain that add to the heavy burden of living with IBS.

How Harmful Are IBS Symptoms?

Experts know that while the symptoms of IBS can hurt every bit as much as those of any other life-threatening disease, they aren't harmful and won't lead to more serious medical problems. IBS won't permanently damage your intestines, or lead to intestinal bleeding or cancer.

Is it IBS . . . or Something Else?

If you've got symptoms of IBS, you probably have spent some time worrying about whether you might have a more serious bowel disease such as ulcerative colitis, Crohn's disease, or stomach or colon cancer.

IBS is quite different from either ulcerative colitis or Crohn's disease, two gastrointestinal (GI) diseases that belong to a group of illnesses called *inflammatory bowel disease* (IBD). Inflammatory disorders occur when the body's immune system attacks its own tissues. For example, rheumatoid arthritis is a common inflammatory condition affecting the lining of multiple joints, usually in the hands and feet. When inflammation affects the lining and wall of the intestine it can trigger a gut reaction, resulting in bowel problems that feel like some IBS symptoms.

While IBS and IBD share similar symptoms of diarrhea and pain, they have very different causes. The symptoms in IBS patients *aren't* caused by inflammation of the bowel but by "faulty wiring" in the network of nerves that carry information between the brain and gut, a point I'll discuss later. While it's possible to have both IBS and IBD, the overwhelming majority of patients have either one or the other. Following are some of the GI diseases with symptoms that mimic IBS.

Crohn's disease In addition to pain often felt in the right side of the abdomen and diarrhea that may be bloody, other symptoms of Crohn's disease include vomiting, low-grade fever, reduced appetite, and weight loss. Crohn's disease can affect any area of the GI tract from the mouth to the rectum, and even the skin on the outside of the anal opening. However, it most commonly affects the lower part of the small intestine, where persistent inflammation spreads deep through multiple layers of tissue of the intestinal wall.

Ulcerative colitis Whereas Crohn's spreads deeply through layers of the GI tract, ulcerative colitis damages only the innermost layer of the colon (the large intestine) and rectum, where inflammation causes bleeding sores (ulcers). The most common symptoms of ulcerative colitis include abdominal pain and often-bloody diarrhea. Unlike IBS, ulcerative colitis causes a progressive inflammation that begins in the rectum and spreads through the colon, leading to rectal bleeding, weight loss, and fever. Ulcerative colitis is often accompanied by physical symptoms not directly related to inflammation in the colon such as eye inflammation, joint pain, skin rashes, and mouth ulcers. Doctors do not know whether these problems are a result or cause of the disease.

Diverticular disease Diverticulosis is a common gut problem characterized by small pouches or sacs that form on the muscle wall of the colon. About 10 percent of Americans over the age of 40 have this condition, which

Potentially Serious Red Flags

Symptoms of abdominal pain and irregular bowel habits can be caused by many conditions besides IBS. The exact cause isn't always clear at first. Some conditions can be serious and life threatening, others aren't. While the symptoms of IBS can be just as painful and disabling as those of more serious disorders, they aren't caused by tissue damage to your gut.

That's why it's important to know whether you have any signs and symptoms of more serious bowel problems caused by significant damage to your gut. These red flags aren't characteristic of IBS, and may mean that you may have a more serious condition that needs medical attention. Schedule an appointment with your doctor if you have any of the following:

- Blood in the stool (blood can appear as red streaks, or make the stool look like black tar)
- A weight loss of approximately seven pounds in a short amount of time with no known reason (such as dieting or exercising)
- A frequent low-grade fever (102°F or lower)
- Symptoms that begin suddenly for the first time after age 50
- Abdominal pain that wakes you up in the middle of the night
- A family history of cancer of the large intestine, an inflammatory bowel disease, or celiac disease
- Sudden shift from normal bowel habits to diarrhea or constipation

If your doctor has diagnosed you with IBS and you have no red-flag symptoms, you should feel relieved knowing you likely don't have a serious disease that is damaging your gut. Some of the symptoms above may still apply to you but shouldn't necessarily cause alarm. For example, while blood in the stool can be a sign of more serious GI problems such as Crohn's disease or colon cancer, it's also a symptom of a bothersome but harmless problem such as hemorrhoids. Similarly, having a strong family history of colon cancer increases the risk of having a more serious GI disease but doesn't necessarily rule out IBS. It's important to discuss any red flag symptoms with your doctor and see whether more extensive evaluation is right for you.

becomes more common as people age. In fact, about half of all people over age 60 have diverticulosis. The condition is believed to be due to eating a low-fiber diet that requires the colon to work harder to move small, hard stool. Over time, strong contractions of the colon push its inner lining outward through gaps in the muscle walls, forming sacs (called *diverticuli*). The sacs themselves don't usually cause bowel problems, although patients might occasionally experience mild cramps, bloating, or constipation. In up to a quarter of people with diverticulosis, the sacs become inflamed or infected, blocking or obstructing the colon. This condition, called *diverticulitis*, may cause pain or tenderness in the left side of the lower abdomen. If infection is the cause of diverticulitis, the pain may be accompanied by chills, fever, nausea and vomiting, cramps, and constipation. The severity of symptoms depends partly on the severity of the infection or inflammation.

Colorectal cancer Cancers that affect either the colon or rectum are called *colorectal* cancer. In most cases, colorectal cancer develops from a small growth called a polyp that develops on the inner wall of the colon or rectum. Sometimes colorectal cancer starts after a cell within the lining of the large intestine becomes cancerous. When colorectal cancer first develops and is small, it does not usually cause symptoms. As it grows, symptoms can vary, depending on where the cancer is. The most common symptoms include bouts of diarrhea and constipation, gas pains, changes in bowel habits, blood (either bright red or very dark) in the stool, paleness and fatigue caused by anemia, stool that looks narrower than usual, lower abdominal pain and tenderness, and weight loss with no known reason.

HOW IS IBS DIAGNOSED?

You probably have been struggling with a variety of symptoms for some time. Even though IBS is a common problem, only a fraction of sufferers ever seek medical help. Once symptoms begin, most IBS patients suffer silently for years before they finally receive a proper diagnosis. Yet it's important to see your doctor if you have a recurring change in the severity, nature, and impact of bowel habits. It's important because your doctor will want to confirm that you have symptoms of IBS, and rule out other more serious GI diseases or conditions that mimic symptoms of IBS, including:

- Ulcerative colitis
- Celiac disease
- Crohn's disease
- Bacterial infections
- Colon cancer
- Endometriosis
- Bowel obstructions
- Thyroid disorder
- Diverticular disease

To find out what's going on with your GI tract, you may choose to visit your primary care physician or a specialist in the treatment of digestive tract diseases (a gastroenterologist). When you go to the appointment, it's important that you clearly and briefly explain your symptoms—no one knows them like you do! You can help your doctor help you by preparing answers to the following questions:

- When did symptoms start?
- How often do they occur?
- How do they make you feel?
- What makes them feel better or worse?
- When do they occur?
- How long do they last?
- How do they affect your life?

Don't be reluctant to describe symptoms that seem embarrassing—your doctor has heard it all before! And don't leave something out because you're worried about taking up too much time. Make sure you leave the doctor's office with answers to all of your concerns or questions. If you don't understand something your doctor says, ask to have it explained again. One way to get the most out of your visit is to read over the list in the box on page 24 and check the boxes that apply to you.

Then bring this list when you meet with your doctor so he or she can better understand your symptoms.

Does This Sound Familiar?

During the past three months, I've experienced the following symptoms:

- ❏ Abdominal pain or discomfort
- ❏ Relief of abdominal discomfort or pain after a bowel movement
- ❏ A change in the frequency of bowel movements—either much more often (diarrhea) or much less frequent (constipation)
- ❏ Stool that is loose and watery, or lumpy and hard
- ❏ Bloated or swollen stomach
- ❏ A strong, sudden urge to go to the bathroom, causing worry that I won't make it in time
- ❏ Straining when having a bowel movement
- ❏ Mucus in the stool
- ❏ A feeling that I haven't fully finished a bowel movement
- ❏ My bowel problems are recurring and keep me from doing everyday things and living my life as I want.

Because there is no specific medical test for IBS, a clear description of your symptoms will give your doctor powerful clues as to whether you have IBS or another GI disease with similar features. In the past, IBS was a "wastebasket" medical diagnosis that physicians used only after they couldn't explain symptoms in any other way. Thanks to recent scientific advances, today an experienced physician can usually diagnose IBS by listening to you describe your symptoms and comparing them to a symptom checklist called the Rome Diagnostic Criteria for IBS. The current version of the Rome criteria—called Rome III—is a classification system that physicians use to determine whether patients have IBS and other functional GI problems. It was developed by an international group of scientists who became frustrated with the inefficient way IBS was being identified.

Diagnosing IBS by first excluding all other possible causes of symptoms is expensive, time-consuming, painful, and frustrating for patients and physicians. Experts reasoned that it would be more efficient and helpful to develop a specific set of diagnostic criteria that identified the specific set of symptoms IBS patients had—not what they didn't have. The Rome III criteria define IBS as abdominal discomfort or pain that occurs for at least three days per month over a three-month span, and that is associated with at least two or more of the following symptoms:

- Pain or discomfort that eases or stops after a bowel movement
- A change in the frequency of bowel movements
- A change in appearance of stool (harder or softer)

Patients who have a diagnosis of IBS also complain of other symptoms. While the Rome III diagnosis of IBS does not require any of the following symptoms, they can strengthen your doctor's confidence that you have IBS.

- Less than three bowel movements a week, or more than three bowel movements a day
- Straining to empty your bowels
- A sudden urge to have a bowel movement or a feeling of not fully emptying your bowels
- Passing mucus in the stool
- Abdominal distension, fullness, or bloating
- Lumpy, hard stool or loose, watery stool

In the vast majority of cases, IBS can be reliably diagnosed based on your description of the pattern and severity of symptoms, a physical exam, your personal medical history, and the Rome criteria, *without* extensive and invasive medical tests. The extent of any further medical evaluation you may undergo will vary depending on the nature of your symptoms, how long you've had symptoms, your age, family history, and what symptoms you describe (or don't describe), when they began, and how they have changed over time. For example, because of the greater incidence of colon cancer in older patients, someone over age 50 whose symptoms are severe and began suddenly may require more extensive medical testing than a younger person whose symptoms developed gradually and persisted for many years.

If your doctor decides on a more complete medical evaluation, he or she will take a complete medical history that includes a careful description of symptoms and do a physical examination. During the examination, your doctor may press deeply on the lower left part of your abdomen and perform a digital rectal examination. This requires the doctor to insert a gloved, lubricated finger into the rectum and check for anything abnormal. While patients with IBS often experience these procedures as mildly uncomfortable, these sensations do not necessarily mean there is something physically wrong with your GI tract. Depending on the nature of your symptoms, age, medical and family history, the doctor may next order a blood or stool test.

Blood Tests

Blood is easy to sample and contains important information about how different parts of your body are working. In most cases, blood tests and a description of your symptoms are enough to confirm whether you have IBS. The most common tests your doctor may order include a CBC (complete blood count, TSH (thyroid stimulating hormone), and ESR (erythrocyte sedimentation rate).

A complete blood count (CBC) assesses the three major types of cells in blood: red blood cells, white blood cells, and "sticky cells" or platelets (the blood count). A shortage of red blood cells can cause a condition called anemia. This can lead to health problems because red blood cells contain a substance called hemoglobin that delivers oxygen to all the cells in the body. Medical causes of anemia include certain rare inherited disorders, infections, nutritional disorders like vitamin or iron deficiency, and serious bowel problems like Crohn's disease. White blood cells are infection-fighting cells that grow and flood your bloodstream when you have an infection or an inflammatory problem. If you have an inflammation or infection, your white blood cell levels may be higher than normal.

Because thyroid disease is common in many young adults who are most likely to develop IBS, your doctor wants to know if your body has the right amount of thyroid hormones by measuring the pituitary hormone TSH. High TSH means your thyroid level is too low, while a low TSH means your thyroid level is too high. Underactivity of the thyroid gland (hypothyroidism) can cause constipation, while an overactive thyroid gland (hyperthyroidism) can cause diarrhea.

An ESR (commonly known as the "sed rate") is a general test of inflammation that measures how quickly red blood cells fall and settle to the bottom of a glass test tube. Normally, red cells fall slowly. Inflammation causes blood cells to descend more rapidly, elevating the sed rate. A sed rate test won't point to the location or reason for inflammation; in any case, inflammation is not a symptom of IBS.

Stool Tests

Because parasites can settle in the GI tract and cause diarrhea, a doctor may give patients with diarrhea-predominant IBS a special kit to collect a stool sample at home. The sample is sent to a lab to check whether parasites or ova (the egg stage of a parasite) are infecting the intestine. In addition, a fecal occult blood test is often performed to detect hidden bleeding from the digestive tract, typically from the stomach, intestine, or rectum.

Blood in the stool is not a symptom of IBS. But even if you have blood in the stool, it doesn't mean you definitely have a serious GI disease. Blood may be caused by hemorrhoids or a slight rectal tear (fissure) in the anus. Anal fissures may occur after a constipated person strains to produce a hard, dry stool during a bowel movement. Both anal fissures and hemorrhoids are treatable and relatively minor digestive health problems.

Your doctor may also want to examine the fat content of your stool. Normally, fat is completely absorbed from the intestine, so that a healthy stool should contain virtually no fat. Some digestive diseases cause excess fat in your stool because the fat isn't digested and absorbed normally by your intestine.

Many IBS experts believe that physicians can confidently arrive at an IBS diagnosis without ordering lots of diagnostic tests. However, for patients with more complicated symptoms and medical histories, more invasive diagnostic testing may be required. These tests may include an upper and lower GI series, colonoscopy or sigmoidoscopy, imaging scans or X-rays, lactose intolerance tests, and/or a celiac antibody screening.

Upper/Lower GI Series

An upper GI test is a set of X-rays that examines the organs of the upper part of the digestive system: the esophagus, stomach, and the first section of the small intestine. Before the test, the patient swallows a metallic-tasting, chalky, liquid called barium, which fills and coats the inside of organs so they show up on an X-ray. The upper GI series can show the location of any narrowing or blockage of the upper GI tract, tumors, ulcers, or a problem with the way an organ is working.

The X-rays of a lower GI series examine the rectum, the large intestine, and the lower part of the small intestine. In this test, a lubricated enema tube is gently injected into the rectum and introduces barium. A barium enema allows abnormalities to appear on an X-ray that may help diagnose several different conditions, such as small growths (polyps) in the lining of the intestine, ulcers, small pouchlike sacs that protrude from the wall of the lining (diverticula), strictures or sites of narrowing and obstruction, IBD, tumors, cancer, and other problems.

Colonoscopy or Sigmoidoscopy

These more direct imaging tests allow for visual and microscopic examination of the intestine. In both tests, the doctor inserts through the anus a long, lighted tube armed with a camera, which transmits images of the colon to a TV monitor. These tests help gauge the severity of inflammation and ulceration as well as how much of the colon is diseased.

A sigmoidoscopy allows your doctor to evaluate the lower third of the colon from the rectum through the sigmoid. The sigmoid colon is almost always inflamed if other parts of your colon are, making this a fairly reasonable screening test for IBD and other inflammatory conditions. With this procedure, a doctor can see bleeding, inflammation, abnormal growths, or early signs of colon cancer. A flexible sigmoidoscopy (a "flex-sig") allows the doctor to look around the twists and turns of your colon better than a rigid sigmoidoscopy. It does not require any sedation, which makes it an easy procedure your doctor can perform right in the office.

A colonoscopy permits the doctor to view the entire large intestine for signs of disease such as cancer of the colon or rectum, inflammation, or polyps (small, cherry-size growths on the inside wall of the large intestine). Although it's most often used to look for early signs of cancer in the colon and rectum, it can be used to identify problems associated with IBD or diverticular disease. A colonoscopy requires extensive preparation, whereby you must clean out your colon for 24 hours prior to the procedure. It also requires something called "conscious sedation," a light form of anesthesia that must be done in a hospital or clinic setting. Polyps can be removed during a colonoscopy, and other small tissue samples can be sent to a lab for a biopsy to spot cancer or other GI disease. If there is bleeding in the colon during the procedure, the physician can inject medication or pass a laser, heater probe, or electrical probe through the scope to stop the bleeding.

A recently developed form of colonoscopy is called virtual colonoscopy (VC). VC uses X-rays and computers to produce two- and three-dimensional images of the colon (large intestine) from the lowest part, the rectum, all the way to the lower end of the small intestine and display them on a screen. VC is more comfortable than conventional colonoscopy for some people because it is not invasive. As a result, no sedation is needed, and patients can return to usual activities or go home after the procedure without the aid of another person. VC provides clearer, more detailed images than a conventional X-ray using a barium enema (lower GI series). It also takes less time than either a conventional colonoscopy or a lower GI series. On the negative side, the doctor cannot take tissue samples or remove polyps during VC, so a conventional colonoscopy must be performed if abnormalities are found. Also, VC does not show as much detail as a conventional colonoscopy, so polyps smaller than 10 millimeters in diameter may not show up on the images.

Doctors recommend that anyone over age 50 have a colonoscopy as part of a routine screening examination to rule out colon cancer. Colonoscopy or sigmoidoscopy also may be recommended in younger patients with a strong family history of colon cancer and certain symptoms (such as diarrhea and weight loss) that may suggest a potentially more serious GI problem such as inflammatory bowel disease.

Computed Tomographic (CT or CAT) Scan

In some cases, your doctor may order a computer-aided X-ray called a computed tomography (CT or CAT) scan of the abdomen. The CT scan takes 3D cross-sectional images of the large and small intestines, stomach, liver, spleen, and diaphragm. These pictures can help identify suspected problems such as tumors, infections, kidney stones, diverticular disease, or appendicitis that may cause symptoms such as pain.

Lactose Intolerance Tests

Patients with lactose intolerance have trouble digesting significant amounts of a milk sugar called lactose, because of a lack of the enzyme lactase. People without this enzyme may have digestive problems that mimic some of the symptoms of IBS, such as nausea, cramps, bloating, gas, and diarrhea. Lactose intolerance can be hard to diagnose based on symptoms alone, because typical symptoms could be caused by many other conditions, including IBS.

Two common methods used to diagnose lactose intolerance are the lactose intolerance and the hydrogen breath tests. During the lactose intolerance test, a patient first fasts and then drinks a liquid containing lactose. Several blood samples are then taken over a two-hour period to measure the person's blood sugar level.

The hydrogen breath test measures the amount of hydrogen in a person's breath. Hydrogen and other gases are released after undigested lactose ferments in the body. The hydrogen is then absorbed into the blood and lungs. Because there is normally very little hydrogen in the breath, a higher level of hydrogen can support a diagnosis of lactose intolerance. However, because foods, medication, and cigarettes can influence hydrogen levels in the body, this breath test is not foolproof.

Celiac Antibody Screening

Some of the symptoms of IBS (diarrhea, cramping, bloating) mimic those of celiac disease, a condition that damages the surface of the small intestine and interferes with absorption of nutrients from food. People who have celiac disease can't tolerate a protein called gluten often found in bread, pasta, cookies, pizza crust, and other foods containing wheat, rye, or barley. Eating these foods makes people with celiac disease very sick because their immune system responds by damaging the small intestine. This is because patients with celiac disease have higher-than-normal levels of certain autoantibodies in their blood. Antibodies are protective proteins the immune system produces in response to substances that the body perceives to be threatening. Autoantibodies are proteins that react against the body's own molecules or tissues.

To screen for celiac disease, physicians will usually make sure the patient is on a gluten-containing diet before measuring celiac-related antibodies in the blood. To confirm the diagnosis, the doctor may obtain tiny tissues from the small intestine to check for damage caused by celiac disease.

WHO GETS IBS?

Because people find the symptoms of IBS so unpleasant and are reluctant to discuss them, it's easy to lose sight of how many people actually have this illness. Experts estimate that up to 20 percent of the world's population suffers from this condition. With 40 million people with IBS in the United States alone, more people suffer from IBS than diabetes, asthma, migraine, or heart disease.

IBS afflicts people from all walks of life, ethnic and racial backgrounds, age groups, and social classes. Although IBS symptoms usually start in late adolescence or early adulthood, many people have the impression that IBS is a young person's problem. In fact, IBS may be much more common among the elderly than once thought. Experts currently estimate that between 10 to 20 percent of the elderly in the general population suffer from undiagnosed IBS. Some physicians may be reluctant to consider IBS as a diagnosis, preferring to focus on other GI problems that are common in the elderly, such as diverticulosis. At the other extreme some physicians regard symptoms of IBS as just a part of getting old. When some elderly patients complain of IBS symptoms, they hear: "You don't have IBS, you just have an old bowel."

One group that is disproportionately affected by IBS is women—

between 60 and 70 percent of all diagnosed IBS patients in the United States are women. This is particularly true for younger women; those between the ages of 15 and 24 show a sharp increase in diagnosis not seen in men of the same age group. Experts aren't sure why more women than men are diagnosed with IBS, but laboratory studies suggest that the biological make-up of the sexes may be one reason. Women report higher pain sensitivity when the colon is stretched. This pain sensitivity is believed to amplify pain signals and cause the intestines to overreact to stimuli. Scientists think pain sensitivity plays an important role in influencing IBS symptoms in 80 percent of patients.

Cultural factors also may help explain gender differences in IBS cases. Some experts believe that IBS is diagnosed more often in women living in Western countries because they are more likely to seek medical treatment for IBS symptoms. It could be that American men may be too embarrassed to seek help for IBS symptoms. An otherwise healthy young man also may be much less likely to see a doctor regularly, when such complaints might be voiced. Most women, on the other hand, see a gynecologist at least once a year, when they have an opportunity to mention GI symptoms and be referred to a GI specialist. However, in some non-Western countries such as India and Sri Lanka, where men are more likely to seek medical help than women, IBS is as common among men as it is in women in Western countries. This suggests that the culture in which we live influences who gets treated for IBS.

Although IBS is diagnosed equally in Caucasians, African Americans, and Hispanics, there appear to be differences in how ethnic groups respond to symptoms. Some studies suggest that Hispanic Americans are less likely to seek medical care for IBS than non-Hispanic Caucasian Americans. Those Hispanics who don't pursue conventional medical options are more likely to turn to traditional folk remedies for relief. African Americans are also less likely to seek medical care for IBS than Caucasians.

SO WHAT CAUSES IBS?

IBS is neither a psychiatric disorder nor associated with tissue damage to the digestive tract, as seen in inflammatory bowel disease. Instead, IBS is considered a *functional disorder*, which means that the bowel doesn't work the way it should, even though medical tests show there's nothing wrong with the physical structure of the bowels. In people with IBS, the nerves and muscles in the bowel are supersensitive to triggers such as certain foods, hormones, or stress. This "irritability" in response to these triggers can cause a wide range of symptoms, including abdominal pain or discomfort and bowel problems.

Scientists believe that a combination of complex factors including heredity, brain patterns, psychological makeup, infection, hormones, and trauma history can play a role in causing IBS. Just how these factors influence IBS varies from one patient to the next.

Motility

Motility refers to the process by which food and waste make their way through the digestive system. Indeed, many IBS patients show abnormal patterns of motility. The time it takes material to pass through the digestive system is called transit time. IBS patients with diarrhea have a shorter transit time than IBS patients with constipation. As a group, however, intestinal transit time varies greatly among IBS patients. This explains why many IBS patients report watery and loose stool one week and hard, lumpy stool the next. Motility also can be measured by the strength and frequency of muscle contractions in the gut. Patients with diarrhea may have stronger, more frequent muscle contractions that pass feces too quickly through the colon to remove enough water to make a solid stool. The result is watery and loose stool. Patients with constipation may have far fewer muscle contractions or may have such strong contractions that feces move too slowly through the gut. This results in hard, difficult-to-pass stool. Between 25 and 75 percent of IBS patients have abnormal motility. However, motility does not necessarily explain pain, incomplete emptying, and bloating. Abnormal motility is also seen in other gut problems so it is not unique to IBS. Nonetheless, motility appears to play a more important role in less severe cases of IBS.

Genes

Does one of your parents, children, or siblings have IBS symptoms? If so, you're not alone. Researchers have discovered that IBS can run in families. In fact, the risk of having IBS nearly doubles in families of people with the disorder, according to Mayo Clinic researchers—this finding suggests that IBS may have a genetic component. Yet scientists doubt IBS is inherited in the same way as hair or eye color. Instead, it's most likely that parents pass on to their children a predisposition or tendency to experience IBS symptoms. When this predisposition is combined with a trigger in the environment, symptoms can develop. Common environmental triggers include a financial setback, trauma, the breakup of a close relationship, a move to a new neighborhood, or the loss of a loved one or job.

Inheriting a predisposition for a problem like IBS doesn't mean that you'll definitely develop IBS. One way of studying the genetic effect of IBS is by studying twins. There are two types of twins: identical and fraternal twins; they differ in the number of genes they share. Identical twins are genetic duplicates of each other—they share all their genes—while fraternal twins share 50 percent of their genes. If IBS had a strong genetic component, we would expect that a large proportion of identical twins would have IBS. This question was studied by researchers at the University of Washington. They found that while having an identical twin doubles the risk of developing IBS, the great majority—more than 80 percent—of twins, either identical or fraternal, don't have IBS. In other words, IBS doesn't necessarily occur in people who are biologically identical. Also, IBS can occur in people who have no family history of the disorder.

This suggests that the genetic factor is only one piece of the larger IBS puzzle. Further, it's unclear whether families are passing on specific genes that "cause" IBS or specific ways of behaving that increase the likelihood of developing IBS. These behaviors may be learned in social environments shared by family members while we are growing up. For example, children listen and watch how parents deal with problems, and then model their own behavior based on these early observations. In this way, overprotective parents may sensitize their children to worry about their own physical symptoms, and fail to teach the type of coping skills that make it easier to manage health problems later in life. Indeed, researchers at Johns Hopkins found that individuals who received lots of sympathy and attention from their mothers when they had bowel symptoms growing up were more likely to develop IBS as adults. In addition, limited or underdeveloped coping skills may explain why children of parents with IBS visit the doctor much more often with IBS symptoms than children whose parents don't have it.

Of course, even if you inherited an IBS gene from your parents it doesn't mean you'll definitely develop IBS yourself. This is because you can always learn techniques for thinking and behaving in ways that prevent IBS symptoms, control symptoms from occurring, or reduce their severity when they occur.

Brain Activity

Normally, the minute-to-minute activity in your digestive system takes place unconsciously and registers in your brain only when your body signals a risk of physical damage to the tissues or internal organs. This is why stomach pain caused by a tainted clam or a ruptured appendix grabs your attention—and why you don't notice the strong, vigorous muscle contractions that help your digestive system operate normally during the day.

While each of us has a different threshold for detecting gut stimuli, IBS patients appear more sensitive to normal gut activities such as muscle contractions, gas bubbles, or passage of stool—activities that often go unnoticed in people without IBS. These findings have led some scientists to speculate that the brain circuits responsible for regulating unpleasant sensations such as gut pain misfire in IBS patients. Indeed, in one study conducted at UCLA, researchers took high-tech brain scans of IBS patients and healthy volunteers as their colons were stretched enough to simulate a mild stomach cramp. This procedure allowed scientists to measure what parts of the brain "light up" when an IBS flare-up occurs.

The scientists discovered that IBS patients showed a distinctive pattern of brain activity when the colon was stretched. People without IBS had more activity in brain regions that help quiet the processing of pain signals. But IBS patients showed activity in the parts of the brain that heighten negative emotions, draw attention to unpleasant sensations, and increase alertness. In other words, healthy volunteers responded to colon pain by activating brain centers that lower the volume of discomfort, while IBS patients responded by tripping an alarm reaction in the brain that magnifies unpleasant gut sensations. Interestingly, research conducted at the University at Buffalo (SUNY) showed that people with IBS who learn to manage and control symptoms using the skills and strategies described in this book can partly reverse these altered brain responses.

Psychological Distress

Because there is no specific physical cause for IBS, it has long been dismissed as a psychological or psychiatric problem. Not true! IBS is simply a problem in how the GI system works. Calling IBS a psychiatric disorder is a bit like calling your car "crazy" when it breaks down.

It's true that 60 percent of IBS patients who consult their physicians at specialized GI clinics suffer from problems with clinical depression, anxiety, or other personal difficulties. But it's important to remember that these studies are based on patients who go to a gastroenterologist for treatment. They don't include the great majority of people with IBS symptoms who don't seek medical attention.

In fact, a series of studies conducted by University of North Carolina researchers found that people with IBS symptoms who don't consult their physicians had psychological profiles that were as normal and free of psychiatric problems as people without bowel symptoms. If IBS was really a psychological problem, you'd expect more distress in people with symptoms, whether or not they sought medical attention. It's very possible that people with IBS reach out for medical help after their symptoms become so bad that their emotional well-being suffers.

This could be one important reason why stress is so important in IBS. In fact, British researchers found that two-thirds of patients with IBS experienced a stressful life event just before their symptoms began. For most people, IBS begins in early adulthood, a time when people experience a barrage of stressful events like leaving home, completing school, becoming financially independent, starting full-time careers, and establishing intimate relationships. Does this make IBS a stress disorder? No. There's no good scientific evidence that psychological stress *causes* IBS—but stress can aggravate its physical symptoms just as it does with other medical conditions like cancer or heart disease. And IBS patients don't have a monopoly on the havoc that stress can throw at the gut. The majority of people without IBS symptoms report that stress can cause bowel symptoms, too. It's just that people with IBS report that the impact of stress on their bowel symptoms is stronger. For these reasons, people with IBS must be more proactive than the average person about managing their stress.

Infection and Bacteria in the Gut

Some experts recently developed the theory that IBS may be caused by excess bacteria (called *bacterial overgrowth*). Bacterial overgrowth refers to a condition in which abnormally large numbers of bacteria are found in the small intestine and resemble the bacteria found in the large intestine. This condition is sometimes referred to as a "leaky gut" and can cause bloating, excess gas, diarrhea, and pain after meals.

In a small study of 100 patients, researchers at the University of Southern California found that about 80 percent of patients with IBS who underwent a specialized breath test exhaled certain gases produced by bacteria in the intestines. Believing that these gases were an indirect measure of bacterial overgrowth, the scientists then treated patients with oral antibiotics, which is a primary treatment for bacterial overgrowth. The researchers found that about half the patients reported many fewer IBS symptoms when they returned for follow-up testing. The researchers concluded that bacteria was causing IBS. While this theory is intriguing, many gastroenterologists believe that bacterial overgrowth is pretty rare (affecting less than 10 percent of IBS patients), and they're reluctant to accept bacteria as a culprit of IBS—or use oral antibiotics as a routine treatment for all IBS patients—until these findings are repeated in higher-quality studies by other researchers.

To date, no virus, bacteria, or parasite has been definitely identified as a direct cause of IBS. Some experts believe that these microorganisms may, under specific environmental conditions, indirectly trigger a gut reaction that causes IBS symptoms. Indeed, some people with IBS recall that their symptoms began after an infection in the lining of the stomach and intestine (gastroenteritis). Gastroenteritis is typically caused by eating food or drinking water tainted by human or animal waste. Bacterial infections caused by food poisoning can overwhelm your body's internal defense system and trigger a brief bout of diarrhea that occurs when your colon secretes salt and water instead of absorbing fluids and nutrients. Diarrhea from food poisoning typically lasts about three days, although it can persist for weeks after the infection ends and the intestine has had a chance to replenish its healthy digestive enzymes.

Although most patients recover from gastroenteritis, up to 25 percent go on to develop full-fledged IBS. Among these patients, it's possible that a microbe may sensitize or trigger gut irritability, causing persistent IBS symptoms. This type of IBS—called post-infectious IBS—is more common in women, those who have longer bouts of diarrhea, and those who experience significant interpersonal stress within four months of the initial infection.

It's possible that infection occurring during stress makes the lining of the gut too porous, interfering with its job of keeping harmful substances from passing through into the body. If this happens, bacteria or viruses may invade the gut and increase both the activity of muscles in the bowel and gut sensitivity. While this may explain the pain and bowel symptoms of IBS patients with post-infectious IBS, it applies to a very small proportion of the overall IBS population.

Hormones

It's quite common for a woman's symptoms to fluctuate during certain times of the menstrual cycle, such as during ovulation, pregnancy, a period, or after menopause. Women with IBS are also more likely to suffer from temporary premenstrual syndrome and painful menstrual periods than women without IBS. Not surprisingly, many women first notice IBS symptoms after their first menstrual period. These findings suggest that fluctuations in the levels of female reproductive hormones may influence IBS.

Hormones are special chemical messengers that travel through the blood, transmitting information and instructions from one set of cells to another. They have a hand in just about every biological process you can think of: immune function, reproduction, growth, sleep, mood, and

GI function. The two main female reproductive hormones are progesterone and estrogen. Animal studies suggest that estrogen may lead to increased gut sensitivity. Progesterone—best known for its role in regulating the menstrual cycle and pregnancy—also acts as a relaxant of the smooth muscles such as the gut. Progesterone and estrogen fall to their lowest levels during the premenstrual cycle, when GI symptoms such as pain, diarrhea, and bloating are at their worse. These data suggest that rapid fluctuations in sex hormones have an important role in menstrually related IBS.

Some researchers have linked menstrual-related changes in IBS symptoms of diarrhea and cramps to the production of prostaglandins, a group of hormonelike messenger substances that contribute to pain, inflammation, and in women, stimulate the uterus to contract to pass menstrual fluid. Women who have painful periods have larger amounts of prostaglandins or are more sensitive to these substances. Half the women with IBS in a recent North Carolina survey linked changes in GI symptoms such as abdominal cramping and bloating to changes in their menstrual periods, compared to only 34 percent of non-IBS women. Moreover, nearly 70 percent of the sample reported IBS symptoms that worsened during their periods.

An alternative way of looking at the role of sex hormones is considering whether the circulation of male hormones somehow protects men from worse IBS symptoms. British researchers found that men with lower levels of the male sex hormone testosterone are more sensitive to pain produced when their colon is stretched in laboratory tests. Unfortunately the way the studies were designed makes it hard to know whether hormonal changes cause IBS symptoms.

Other researchers have examined how hormones produced in the GI tract may account for IBS symptoms. Cholecystokinin (CCK) is one gut hormone the small intestine produces that is altered in patients with IBS. CCK influences a number of gut activities; it can slow down how fast food moves through your stomach, increase muscle contractions in the colon, and help secrete its digestive juices. CCK is also what gives you a full feeling after eating a meal. Some researchers believe that worsening symptoms after eating may be due to an exaggerated release of CCK, although research is not conclusive.

Abuse

Sexual and physical abuse are often viewed as critical to the development and persistence of IBS. These findings suggest that while there appears to be a consistent relationship between abuse and subsequent development of medical symptoms, it's probably not specific to IBS. Between 30 and 50 percent of people with IBS symptoms who seek medical attention report a prior history of traumatic events, such as childhood abuse, neglect, or loss of a parent, according to research conducted by many different scientists. By comparison, the rates of child sexual abuse in the general population typically range from 5 percent for men to 20 percent for women. A prior history of abuse among IBS patients has been linked to more severe symptoms, worse quality of life, and the need for more complicated treatment. Does a reliable, consistent association between IBS and abuse mean that abusive experiences *cause* IBS? Probably not.

First, many adults who were abused during childhood often flourish against all odds, showing a remarkable resilience and capacity to convert early life adversity into coping skills that buffer them from developing health problems later in life. The connection between abuse and IBS may not be as strong at it appears, since studies supporting the IBS-abuse relationship are based on patients from GI clinics that don't include people with IBS symptoms who don't seek medical care, most of whom have never been abused.

Second, any role abuse plays in the development of IBS is probably limited. A history of abuse is likely to increase the risk of developing a range of health problems in general and not IBS in particular. This is because the rate of childhood sexual abuse does not appear much higher among those with IBS than among those who later develop other physical or emotional health problems. For example, patients with headache, back pain, pelvic pain, anxiety, depression, and other personal difficulties also report high rates of abuse. These findings suggest that while there appears to be a consistent relationship between abuse and subsequent development of medical symptoms, it's probably not specific to IBS.

Third, research claiming a relationship between IBS and abuse comes from studies that rely on what happened to a group of people in the past. These studies are limited because people may not accurately remember abuse histories. But even carefully designed studies that followed patients over time have not supported a causal relationship between childhood abuse and the development of painful medical conditions that coexist with IBS during adulthood. Generally speaking, this relationship is modest, if it exists at all. Further research is needed to see whether this pattern of findings applies to IBS patients who have a positive history of abuse.

✳

As you can see, there's no single cause of IBS. For some people, physical factors such as genes or an intestinal infection may be the culprit; for others, it may be behavioral and physical factors such as stress, trauma, parenting style, or early life experiences. Most likely, a number of factors work together to explain why you developed IBS.

But it's important to know that when medical problems are chronic, the factors that caused initial symptoms to occur in the first place typically differ from those that keep symptoms continuing. Regardless of how bowel problems started, this book will help you identify and tackle the factors that maintain your symptoms in the long term. To get started, it helps to understand the inner workings of the digestive system in people with and without IBS.

HOW YOUR GI SYSTEM WORKS

Digestion is the process by which food is broken down into small parts so the body can use them to nourish cells and provide energy. The digestive tract begins in the mouth and ends some 30 feet later at the rectum.

Here's how it all works: After you take a bite of an apple, it travels from your mouth to the esophagus, where waves of muscular contractions push food down and into the stomach. Once the chewed food reaches the stomach, it's churned with gastric juices to form a thick liquid. Muscles then move the mixture into the small intestine, a 21-foot tube coiled up in your abdomen that connects the stomach to the large intestine. In the center of your small intestine, food is further broken down and converted to vitamins, minerals, carbohydrates, fats, proteins, and water, which are absorbed through the small intestinal wall into the bloodstream. What's left is a watery mix that's propelled into the colon, where remaining water, salts, and minerals are absorbed. The colon solidifies the remaining material—the stool—before it is pushed into the rectum, where it's stored until you're ready to have a bowel movement.

Food moves through the intestines by a rhythmic, wavelike pattern of muscle contraction and relaxation. This process—remember, it's called motility—is controlled by nerves and hormones, and by electrical activity in the colon muscle. A few times each day, strong muscle contractions move down the colon, pushing waste ahead of them. Some strong contractions result in a bowel movement. In normal individuals, these contractions are rhythmic, neither too fast nor too slow. People with IBS, however, have gut muscles that under certain situations may be more sensitive, speeding up or slowing down the movement of water and waste materials through the colon.

Diarrhea occurs when muscle contractions moving food through the digestive tract become stronger and more frequent. In this case, waste moves through the colon so quickly that there isn't time for the colon to remove enough water from the waste to make a solid stool. The result: a loose, watery stool. These vigorous colon contractions can also cause severe cramps.

Constipation happens when the muscles contract *less* often, so that waste moves too slowly through the colon. Because the waste lingers in the colon, there's more time for fluids to be absorbed, making stools hard and lumpy. When this happens, the muscles in the colon aren't stimulated to contract, and gas can build up and stretch the colon, causing pain.

While changes in the muscular contractions of the colon help explain why some people develop some IBS-related bowel problems, they can't explain other aspects of IBS. For example, the amount of pain you feel doesn't necessarily go hand in hand with the amount of muscle activity in the gut. Even when motility problems are observed, they aren't necessarily accompanied by other symptoms, such as constipation or the urge to defecate. Some people with IBS don't have spasms at all during painful flare-ups. When spasms do occur, they don't always cause symptoms.

Keep in mind that even healthy individuals without IBS can experience intestinal spasms from time to time. Moreover, people with IBS can experience pain in response to normal events, such as having gas in the intestines, eating a small meal, or having a full rectum. This suggests that people with IBS are more sensitive to pain and other unpleasant sensations in their bowels.

THE BRAIN-GUT CONNECTION

The brain plays an important role in how much pain you feel from a given physical stimuli. For this reason, many IBS researchers have turned their focus from strictly the gut to how the brain and gut work together to influence symptoms. Ideally, the brain and the gut work together in a coordinated manner, much like two riders on a tandem bike: The gut sends information to the brain, and signals from the brain are relayed back to the gut. This "cross talk" between the brain and gut is the reason why the smell of a juicy hamburger stimulates secretions in the stomach long before you take your first bite. As long as the brain and gut are communicating in a coordinated way, the body carries out its digestive duties without a hitch.

However, sometimes communication between the brain and gut is disrupted. When communication breaks down repeatedly, the nerve fibers in the gut carrying sensory messages become more sensitive, the colon begins to spasm after only mild stimulation, and the brain loses some of its ability to filter out unwanted pain signals transmitted from the gut. This breakdown in the brain-gut connection can crank up the volume on pain signals so that normal amounts of gas or routine activities in the GI tract that aren't ordinarily perceived as uncomfortable (such as normal stool moving along the colon, or gas) are experienced as painful. Several laboratory studies have found that when a small balloon is inflated in the rectum to simulate abdominal cramping and subjects are asked to rate their level of pain, IBS patients report pain at much lower balloon pressures and volumes that than those that cause pain in healthy volunteers. Scientists refer to this phenomenon as *visceral sensitivity* and regard it as an example of the brain-gut breakdown in action. What causes this breakdown in brain-gut communication? As anyone who has ever felt "butterflies" before going onstage knows, stress is one thing that can disrupt the communication between the brain and gut.

Stress and IBS: Is There a Connection?

Everyone talks about stress these days—how it affects your sleep, blood pressure, bone growth, memory, appetite, sex drive, thyroid, heart, and just about every other part of your body. It should come as no surprise that stress also affects the digestive system.

The colon has lots of nerves that connect it to the brain, and it's also partly controlled by the autonomic nervous system (ANS), an involuntary system of nerves that controls organs such as the heart, stomach, and intestines. An important job of the ANS is the regulation of digestion and the muscle contractions that eliminate solid waste. The autonomic nervous system also controls how we respond physically to stress.

While stress doesn't cause IBS, it can certainly aggravate bowel symptoms. Stress can make food pass through the digestive system very fast and magnify gut sensations. Over time, your bowel can be increasingly sensitive to even small amounts of anxiety or stress. Most people with IBS who carefully track their symptoms can link many flare-ups to an increase in stressful events. *Stress isn't a sign of weakness, mental illness, or inability to handle difficult situations; it's simply how the brain and body react to anything that upsets its regular balance.* The box below lists common ways the body and brain respond to stress.

Body
- Rapid heartbeat
- Sweaty palms
- Faint or dizziness
- Chest pain
- Shortness of breath
- Stomach problems
- Skin rash
- Teeth grinding
- Restless sleep
- Muscle aches
- Exhaustion
- Headaches
- Shakes, chills, hot flashes

Brain
- Procrastination
- Demoralization
- Pessimism
- Worry
- Nervousness, edginess
- Short fuse
- Feeling down
- Memory problems
- Careless mistakes

Stressful events can be negative or positive, big or small. Major stressors are pretty easy to spot. The death of a loved one, losing a job, and going through a divorce are all examples of life events that are obviously stressful. But did you know that positive events such as getting a promotion, buying a new home, having a baby, getting married, or taking a vacation can be just as stressful? Even everyday events or hassles can be just as stressful: the pressure of getting dinner on the table, meeting a deadline, losing your keys, juggling family and work demands, or burning the toast. Because these events seem so minor, you may not realize how they can get under your skin. However, over time the stress they create can build up. You may not notice the gradual increase in your stress level until your stomach acts up.

To understand how stress triggers IBS symptoms, it's important to understand that stress isn't necessarily bad. Sometimes we seek out stress— a scary movie, whitewater rafting, a roller coaster ride, a murder mystery— just for the thrill of it!

The right amount of stress can bring out the best in us. However, too little stress and we feel bored; too much stress and we feel burned out. The proper balance of stress is important for us to perform at our best. For these reasons, it may be helpful to think of stress as the tension on the strings of a violin or guitar. You need just enough to make good music: Too much tension and the strings snap, too little, and there's no music.

How Your Body Reacts to Stress

Back when your caveman ancestor first stumbled out of his cave, his body's ability to respond to stress helped him fend off predators using a kind of physical "alarm system" to stay alive. Hearing the roar of a saber-toothed tiger, the caveman's brain instantaneously triggered the release of adrenaline, which flooded the bloodstream, mobilizing his body to either stand its ground and fight, or flee and retreat. Scientists call this alarm reaction the *fight-or-flight response*. During the fight-or-flight response, physical activities not critical to surviving immediate danger are switched off: Blood in the arms and legs is diverted to support the heart and major muscles, temperature in the hands and feet falls, and digestion screeches to a halt.

If a 300-pound tiger was chasing the caveman, the caveman's most pressing task would be to find a secure cave to hide, not to digest that morning's mastodon steak. After all, the digestive process takes away lots of energy from the muscles, which are needed to fight or flee, and adds a couple of pounds of deadweight stored in the intestines when you need to react as swiftly as possible. To ensure that no resources are wasted on digestion, the body may lighten its load by emptying the digestive tract through defecation. But for another caveman with the mountain lion snapping at his heels, an immediate bathroom break can spell trouble. In this situation, the digestive systems may switch gears and bottle up waste— hence constipation—long enough to reach a safe pit stop.

As you can see, stress turns off nonessential tasks and turns on other emergency responses critical to self-survival:

- Breathing quickens as the lungs take in more oxygen.
- Heart rate and blood pressure increase.
- Muscles tense.
- Perspiration increases.
- The liver releases glucose (sugar) for a quick jolt of energy.
- Blood vessels narrow to reduce bleeding.
- The brain releases endorphins, the body's natural painkiller.

These changes prime the entire body to either fight or run away. When the emergency is over, the fight-or-flight response immediately shuts off and the body downshifts to its normal, non-emergency state. Once the saber-toothed tiger lumbers away and the threat passes, your prehistoric ancestor would calm down and go back to the comfort of his cave.

This alarm reaction was designed in our earliest history to prepare us for short-lived situations of life and death. Those whose bodies were best able to respond to life-threatening situations survived. Those with weaker systems perished. Today, we live in a world that has eliminated most of the physical dangers that stalked our ancestors. In most cases, we can drive down the interstate without worrying that a gang of pirates will hijack our car, or walk down Main Street without thinking that a lion will take us home for lunch. Thanks to modern technological advances, we've conquered most real physical dangers faster than our bodies have been able to adjust. While the threats for our ancestors included grizzly bears and poisonous snakes, today's stress is less physical and more psychological—the criticism of an angry boss, long lines at the checkout counter, that idiot who cut us off on the exit ramp. Today, ordinary stress comes from the pressure of things we can't control, not physical dangers. Yet your brain doesn't make a distinction between everyday hassles and actual physical dangers: It reacts the same way in both cases. When you experience psychological stress, the brain triggers a "false alarm," which sets in motion the fight-or-flight response that is ideally reserved for physical dangers. This explains why you may have had a diarrhea attack when you were scared, or rumblings in your stomach before making a speech.

Unfortunately, today's stress is not an occasional, five-minute fight for survival, but a nonstop series of daily pressures. In fact, experts estimate that today, the average person's fight-or-flight system switches on and off 30 to 50 times daily, compared to just once or twice daily for our cavemen cousins who lived in much more physically dangerous times.

Research shows that repeated activation of the fight-or-flight response, which is built to protect the body from brief physical dangers in the short run, can cause wear and tear on your body when it is triggered on and off over a long time. False alarms can lead to physical problems such as muscle aches, headaches, stomach problems, chest pains, depression, and diabetes. Long-term stress stemming from job or family problems can even increase your chances of catching a cold by weakening your immune system. If these symptoms sound familiar, you should know that you aren't alone. Experts estimate that medical conditions aggravated by stress account for 75 percent of all visits to physicians.

How Your Brain Reacts to Stress

Stress affects not just your body, but also your brain. During brief bursts of stress triggered by physical danger, the brain's capacity to focus and store important information increases. Scanning the environment for signs of a threat or challenge is a real plus when the stress is short-lived and a real physical danger lurks. Brief periods of stress may actually improve memory by helping us remember places to avoid where we faced physical danger.

When stress is continuous, it can cause changes in brain circuits so that memory suffers. Chronic stress also dampens your ability to think clearly, so you're more easily distracted and unable to concentrate. When your body overreacts, you can become on edge, keyed up, hyperalert. When this happens, you may find yourself preoccupied with regrets, frustrations, and misfortunes in the distant past that you wish hadn't happened, or envisioning bad things in the future. Sometimes it's hard to stop those thoughts from occurring, which only adds to your frustration. When you worry, you can lose your sense of perspective. You may spend so much time worrying that you have trouble focusing, functioning at your best, or getting on with life. You may find yourself thinking the worst or jumping to conclusions no matter what the situation. This is most likely to happen when you're facing the unknown and don't have as much control as you'd like. Stress can also hinder your ability to think flexibly and solve problems that require choosing one of many possibilities.

ARE YOU A GUT RESPONDER?

So why do some people get IBS symptoms while others stay healthy?

Remember, IBS is not caused by stress. Having IBS doesn't mean that you're any more stressed out or anxious than other people. We each have a unique way of responding to stress. Some people have a stronger emotional response, becoming irritable, frustrated, or nervous. Stress triggers nervous behavior in some people, such as pacing, tapping, stammering, talking too fast, nail biting, fidgeting, or restlessness. Others respond to stress physically with higher blood pressure, fatigue, muscle tension, headaches, or gastrointestinal problems.

People whose bowel symptoms flare up during stressful situations are called *gut responders*. Of course, you don't have to be diagnosed with IBS to be a gut responder. Two out of every three people *without* IBS report that psychological stress causes the same changes in bowel functioning described by those who *do* have IBS. However, the difference between "healthy" individuals and people with IBS is not the *type* of stress response, but how *long* and how *strong* the stress response is.

If you're like most people with IBS, your symptoms themselves cause stress, which may lead to subsequent changes in how your body reacts to material in the bowel. These changes can worsen symptoms and disrupt your daily life, which in turn can drag you down and cause even more strain. Before long, you're trapped in a vicious circle of bowel symptoms, physical changes, and stress. At the same time, coping with symptoms that occur where and when you least expect becomes more and more difficult.

As symptoms persist, most people struggle to piece together a normal life. But even life's simple pleasures—a walk in the park, a dinner celebration with friends, intimacy, a drive through the countryside—require the planning of a military ground strike.

The good news is that if you can learn how to control stress, you can control your IBS symptoms. In the next chapters, you'll read how more than 20 years of research has shown that behavioral methods can help you control the complex interaction between the brain and the bowel in IBS.

WHAT'S NEXT?

Fortunately, there's hope. Now that you understand what physical and mental changes aggravate IBS, you're ready to start learning what you can do to control them. By following this 10-step program, your symptoms should decrease and your quality of life should improve. You'll find that your confidence in your ability to control symptoms will spill over into other areas of your life, making it easier to bounce back from adversity during everyday life.

The next chapter is an overview of our simple plan to help you reverse this vicious circle by learning new ways of thinking and discovering specific tools to reduce the stress that aggravates bowel symptoms. Approximately 70 percent of the patients who have followed this plan have experienced improvements in symptoms. So read on to learn a new way to finally take control of your bowel symptoms.

HOW THE PLAN WORKS

Linda is a 42-year-old housewife who suffered from severe IBS symptoms, struggling every day with painful knots in her stomach and constipation. "I felt incredible strain from those symptoms," she recalls, and her inability to control them was affecting every area of her life. What was even worse, doctors weren't able to identify a physical cause. "That just sent me over the edge," she says. "I had been to I don't know how many doctors and I was taking a shopping list of drugs and supplements. Nothing worked."

Finally, out of desperation, she turned to the IBS treatment program at the University at Buffalo. A self-admitted skeptic, Linda found it hard to imagine how a nondrug approach could help ease her IBS when all those doctors and medications could not. But because nothing else had worked, she figured she had nothing to lose. "I figured, what the heck!" she says. "I wasn't able to deal with life the way things were."

Within a month after starting the program, she noticed that her symptoms began to improve as she applied the skills she learned. Today, Linda has largely put her symptoms behind her. "I used to take a slew of meds daily. Nothing worked. Now I don't feel any churning in my stomach at all. If I get overwhelmed, I ask myself: 'What can I do to control my symptoms?' Now I'm more aware of how my body responds to things, so if I can't calm down, I ask myself how I want to handle this situation, and then I do it. I would say I'm almost symptom free . . . it's incredible. It's wonderful to know I'm not crazy."

Linda is one of the 40 million Americans living with IBS. Yet sadly, there's no magic pill or dietary remedy that *cures* IBS. The truth is that while medications or diet may ease some IBS complaints for some people, there's no single medication or food that takes care of *all* the symptoms. Medications have had an especially disappointing track record for people with severe IBS, and many carry unpleasant side effects. What too many people never know is that there's a simpler, safer way to gain control of IBS symptoms.

Backed by 20 years of quality research at the State University of New York (SUNY) in both Albany and Buffalo, and years of firsthand clinical experience, the self-management plan that we describe in this book has already helped patients just like you. The key is following this simple 10-step plan aimed at reducing physical tension with muscle relaxation exercises, while easing mental tension by changing the way you think about and solve problems more efficiently. About 70 percent of patients who follow this program learn to improve their symptoms within two months of starting treatment.

Unfortunately, because so few clinics specialize in the behavioral treatment of IBS, many people don't receive the care they deserve. The few who do have access to specialized care feel uncomfortable talking about their symptoms with a doctor. What's worse, all too often, when patients do mention their difficulties, their concerns are dismissed as "nothing to worry about." They're told they should "just live with it."

Of course, if managing IBS was simply a matter of "living with it," you'd have done that long ago! Nobody *wants* to suffer with IBS. There's no reason why you should have to—because taking control of IBS is as simple as understanding what triggers your symptoms, and then developing specific skills to control the symptoms and prevent flare-ups. That's exactly what this book will help you do.

Seem too good to be true? That's understandable. You've probably struggled with your symptoms for years. In fact, nearly half the people with IBS have had symptoms for at least 10 years, according to a recent survey conducted by the International Foundation for Functional GI Disorders. You've probably consulted a number of doctors, undergone lots of tests, altered your diet, and tried all kinds of medications and over-the-counter treatments—all without adequate relief. Why should a nondrug program work any better than all the other pills, potions, and remedies you've tried in the past?

If you think about it, self-care strategies are used very successfully by patients with other chronic illnesses such as asthma, diabetes, and high blood pressure. These illnesses, just like IBS, aren't completely curable, but people can improve their symptoms by learning specific skills to manage the conditions. For example, you can make high blood pressure worse by smoking cigarettes, eating salty food, and not getting enough exercise. You can learn to lower your blood pressure by changing your behavior—getting more exercise, avoiding salty foods, and throwing away your cigarettes. We'll apply this same self-help approach to controlling some of the behaviors that aggravate IBS. Remember, the very same program that you'll read about in this book has already helped many patients in the SUNY Buffalo research program control their IBS symptoms. It worked for them, and it can work for you, too.

Our team has completed more than 20 years of clinical studies that have systematically tested the treatment procedures described in this book. These studies demonstrate that behavioral methods can be effective in treating IBS. Of course, everyone has a unique background, personality, life experiences, and physical and psychological makeup. We can't guarantee that this program will cure your symptoms. But there are solid reasons to believe that if you follow the program and practice the exercises, you'll likely see a significant improvement in your symptoms just like hundreds of patients in the United States, Canada, Germany, Australia, England, and Sweden, have already demonstrated.

Of course, achieving substantial improvement doesn't guarantee that you will get rid of bowel problems permanently. After all, bowel problems are so common that they're really a normal part of life. But patients who learn and carefully practice these skills usually find that the relief they get allows them to live a more comfortable, normal lifestyle.

The research described in this book has helped change the way doctors think about managing IBS. Doctors now know that some of the most powerful treatments for IBS don't come in a pill and can't be eliminated from or added to your diet. That's right—*the single most important factor in controlling your IBS symptoms is YOU!* By following the proven strategies in this book, most people with IBS in our program can dramatically reduce their symptoms as much as by half. So what can you do? Actually, quite a lot.

If you have IBS, you're probably all too aware of the effect it can have on your life. Ask yourself this question: Do you control your bowel symptoms, or do they control you like millions of others? It's time for you to stop being a statistic! You're about to begin a program that will help you understand IBS, control your symptoms, and reclaim your life—all without relying on drugs or dietary changes.

You learn new things all the time: how to use a new computer program, set your DVD, change a flat tire. But few people are ever taught how to manage a chronic illness such as IBS. Most people manage their symptoms by turning to whatever knowledge and skills they may have picked up along the way. Can you imagine using a computer if no one ever taught you how to log on? Programming your DVD without an instruction manual? Forget about it!

Many people learn the hard way that managing IBS well takes more than common sense—you really need to learn a specific set of skills described in this book. The strategies you'll learn are accepted by IBS experts as some of the few clinically proven options for IBS. While there is no fix for IBS, our goal is to teach you these skills so you can gain control over your symptoms and get on with your life.

YOU CAN MANAGE IBS!

In this book, you'll learn how to make simple lifestyle changes to manage your symptoms by following this natural, risk-free, and inexpensive plan. I should explain right up front that we're not going to be changing *you*.

Nobody can tell you what to do. Nobody can *make* you change. Our goal is to give you the road map that other people have used to control their bowel symptoms.

The First Step

It's a lot easier to pop a pill than sit down and learn a set of new skills—but learning new skills is the best way that we have right now to control IBS. To make this program work for you, you'll need to decide if you're ready to make some changes.

- Are you fed up with being controlled by your bowel symptoms?
- Do you want to take charge of your bowel symptoms?
- Are you willing to make some changes in your daily routine to reclaim your life?
- Do you have the motivation to put forth your best effort?
- Do your IBS symptoms make you feel like a prisoner in your body?

If you answered yes to these questions, this book is for you! You'll find that the time and effort it takes to learn these lessons is not nearly as tough as you think—and it's a small price to pay for improving your physical well-being. It's important to understand exactly why you're seeking treatment, because what you hope to get out of treatment will help keep you motivated. Having a strong commitment to change can carry you through rough patches when your symptoms flare up and your goal of IBS relief seems like more trouble than it's worth.

There are many reasons that prompt people to seek help. Here are some of the most common reasons:

- I want to increase my control over my body and life.
- I want to feel better about myself.
- I want to eat what I want.
- I want to improve my social life.
- I want to stop feeling so ashamed about my symptoms.

- I want to improve my work performance (like getting to work on time).
- I want to save money on nutritional supplements, medications, or co-pays.
- I want to decrease pain.
- I want to travel without worrying about where the closest bathroom is.
- I want to feel more at ease.
- I want to feel less pressure from others to do something about my symptoms.
- I want to stop living life between bowel flare-ups.

Do any of these sound like you? Are there others you can think of? Jot down as many reasons you can think of for why you'd like to control your IBS. Some people who get the most out of our program like to keep their list nearby—on the nightstand, in a wallet or purse—to remind them why they want to continue the program. This can strengthen your motivation and increase the likelihood of success when the going gets rough.

HOW THE PLAN WORKS

Our research has identified three keys to this treatment: knowledge, motivation, and skills. You've already gained knowledge by learning more about IBS in the first chapter, and the fact that you opened this book suggests you're motivated to change. If you're reading these pages, it's because your symptoms have not responded as well as you would have liked to conventional medical treatments such as modifying your diet or taking pills.

As you will see, each of the 10 steps in this program focuses on a new skill proven effective for helping people with IBS control their bowel symptoms. You should try to master one step a week before moving on to the next one. Remember, my goal is for you to learn ways to control IBS— not how to speed-read this book.

The 10 steps to this plan are:

Step 1. What's Going On in Your Life?

Step 2. Taking Control of Your Body with Relaxation Skills

Step 3. Applying Relaxation Skills to Everyday Life

Step 4. Outsmart IBS by Tracking Your Thoughts

Step 5. Learning to Think More Constructively

Step 6. Bouncing Back from Adversity

Step 7. Putting Your Thinking Skills Together

Step 8. Solving Problems Efficiently

Step 9. Challenging Core Beliefs

Step 10. Identifying Skills that Work for You

You may find that one skill is more helpful to you than another. If one strategy doesn't tackle your problems, don't get discouraged. The key is having a menu of choices from which to pick. Just like at a restaurant, the larger the menu, the more likely you'll find something that agrees with you. This 10-step plan focuses on controlling IBS by teaching these simple skills:

- Tracking your symptoms, their triggers, and your reactions
- Controlling physical tension
- Thinking constructively
- Solving life's problems efficiently

The first steps focus on relaxing. Of course, knowing how to relax is more than just plopping into a hammock with a glass of lemonade. You'll learn how to help slow down the pace of your body and promote a state of general calmness that's conducive to digestive health. By learning relaxation skills for everyday situations, you'll understand how to detect tension before it reaches a point that can aggravate bowel symptoms.

In the next steps, you'll work on mastering thinking and problem-solving skills to help you target tension triggered by the way you think in high-pressure situations. As you'll see, people with IBS tend to overinterpret negative events, set extremely high (and often unrealistic) standards for themselves, blame themselves for things that go wrong, and underestimate their ability to cope with bad events when they do occur.

Research shows that negative beliefs can affect muscle tension, brain chemistry, blood flow, and bowel function. Negative thoughts also can color the way you look at the world, so that you give up more readily in the face of adversity. You'll learn how to test the usefulness and accuracy of self-defeating thinking patterns and replace them with more helpful ways of thinking. You'll also learn a step-by-step model for problem solving around realistic stressors that can worsen bowel problems. As your skills improve, you'll find you can strengthen your ability to cope with stress and deal more constructively with difficult situations.

Becoming an IBS Expert

This isn't some unrealistic plan we dreamed up out of the blue. Plenty of my patients, just like you, have already gone through the program successfully. You too can succeed with this program if you play an active role in managing your own IBS symptoms. People who benefit most are those who try lots of different ways to manage their symptoms. Pills don't work if you don't take them, and neither will the skills you'll learn if you don't take time to practice them.

In this program, you'll practice how to manage your symptoms at home, during situations where your symptoms occur and you need help the most. This will make it easier to halt your symptoms early, before they become bigger problems.

A home-based program is also convenient — you won't need to travel to the doctor as much, and you'll have more freedom and flexibility to learn and practice skills where the problem occurs. You can progress at your own pace in the comfort of your home as you follow the steps in this book.

You can refer to it at any time, referring to special sections if you get stuck later on and need to get back on track.

WHAT'S NEXT?

Now that you have an overview of the plan, it's time to get started. Part Two of the book takes you through the 10 steps that will help you relieve your IBS symptoms.

PART TWO

A 10-STEP PLAN
FOR SYMPTOM
RELIEF

Equipped with a clearer understanding of IBS, now you are ready to gain control of IBS by learning simple, effective techniques that zero in on the self-defeating behaviors and thoughts that aggravate symptoms. The chapters in Part Two will guide you through the 10 steps of our treatment plan, which is backed by 20 years of solid research with people like you. Each chapter focuses on a specific skill, explains how each skill tackles certain aspects of IBS, provides clear, step-by-step instructions for mastering skills specific to your needs, and gives troubleshooting tips for working around problems that you may face. Because each chapter builds upon the one before it, your skills and confidence in your ability to manage IBS symptoms should increase as you work through the book. User-friendly worksheets, interactive exercises, self-assessment checklists, personal diaries for tracking symptoms and trigger foods, and examples drawn from IBS patients who have successfully completed our program, are included to help you master each skill. The last step is a review of what techniques in your personalized treatment plan worked best and strategies for how to maintain your gains and prevent the symptom flare-ups.

STEP 1

WHAT'S GOING ON IN YOUR LIFE?

Charlene woke up in the morning with a sense of dread before she'd even tossed back the covers. She was giving a big presentation to the Kansas City head office today, and she wanted things to go just right. But she couldn't find her favorite suit, and her shoes were scuffed. The twins started bickering about who could eat the last muffin as the dishwasher started making a funny thumping sound before grinding to a halt. The milk was sour, the dog stepped in his water bowl, and the mail was piling up on the desk in the kitchen. On the way to school, Charlene noticed the gas gauge near "E" at about the time one of the twins spilled milk on the car seat. As rush hour traffic started to back up, Charlene remembered she'd left an important document at home on her bedside table. The day had scarcely begun, and a knot was growing deep in her belly.

Does any of this sound familiar? We all figure we know how destructive the major life stressors can be—divorce, death of a loved one, losing a job, serious illness. But most of us aren't aware of how the daily hassles of modern life can get under our skin and affect our health. A spat with your spouse, a missed deadline, being late for work, getting a parking ticket, losing your keys, or popping a button right before an important meeting— all these things can build up and become more upsetting than many more "significant" problems. Trying to balance work, home, friends, and family can pile one small stress on top of another. Taken all together, they can pack a significant punch to your physical and mental health.

"Oh, sure," you're probably saying. "I'm under lots of pressure at work, and I don't get enough help around the house. Of course I'm stressed! Wouldn't everyone feel the same way?"

Maybe so, but if you have IBS, those daily hassles aren't going to help your symptoms. You need to take a really close look at exactly what's going on with your life. If you're reading this book, you already know you have IBS and you probably have a pretty good idea that you need help to manage some of your stress. That's why the first step in our IBS 10-step treatment plan is designed to help you tease out exactly what hassles trip you up, and how they affect you. This is important, because if you don't know exactly where the strain is coming from you can't fix it. And if you can link your bowel problems to certain triggers, you'll begin to see your problems as predictable and therefore controllable.

Top 10 Daily Hassles

A recent survey of American adults identified their top 10 daily stresses:

1. Weight worries
2. Family members' health
3. Rising prices
4. Home maintenance
5. Too many things to do
6. Misplacing or losing things
7. Yard work
8. Money worries
9. Crime
10. Physical appearance

TRACK YOUR SYMPTOMS

Stress isn't the only thing we want you to really understand. It's also important to figure out exactly what symptoms you have, and when and what triggers them. You may say: "Oh, I always get a bout of IBS when I eat French fries and drink coffee." But some days this may happen, and other days it might not. And then sometimes your symptoms may just seem to come out of nowhere.

"My IBS is so weird," 45-year-old Karen says. "I can eat a burger and fries six times a month, and five times I'll be fine. The sixth time I'll get explosive diarrhea minutes after eating a burger. Then, the other day I hadn't eaten anything and the next thing you know, I had a serious flare that came totally out of the blue." There probably was a very good reason for Karen's "mysterious" flares, but she wasn't paying enough attention to notice what it was.

Tracking all your symptoms for at least a two-week period will help you pinpoint exactly what symptoms you have and give you valuable clues into what's really triggering them. Because there isn't a simple cure for IBS, controlling this problem requires your active participation. If you have IBS, the task of monitoring and regulating bowel function is more than your body can do on its own. For this reason, it's important for you to keep a log of your symptoms. So many variables can affect bowel symptoms:

- What and when you eat
- Daily hassles
- Illness
- Attitude
- Activities
- Schedule changes
- Hormone fluctuations

Monitoring symptoms may feel like a bit of a hassle at first, but you'll be surprised how soon it'll become second nature as its value becomes more obvious. We have yet to meet a person whose lifestyle makes monitoring truly impossible! Of course, you're more likely to keep accurate records if you know why it's so important. Here's why you'll want to do a good monitoring job:

- *Monitoring reveals important information about your symptoms.* You may think you're all too familiar with your bowel symptoms, but there are probably some aspects that may not be so obvious. Tracking your symptoms will help you identify more subtle triggers of your symptoms and how you respond to them. Keeping tabs on your symptoms can reveal patterns that you might not have been aware of, so that you can target them with the self-management skills you will learn.

- *Monitoring helps you change.* Knowing that symptoms often have a predictable pattern creates opportunities for change and improvement. This plays a big part in altering habits and can lead to dramatic changes in how you feel. As you become more skilled in tracking your bowel symptoms, you'll recognize that flare-ups don't always come up out of the blue. Careful monitoring helps you see that symptoms are often part of a chain of events triggered by an often predictable set of specific situations, thoughts, sensations, and behaviors. Not all symptoms are easy to track back to specific events, but we want you to get a handle on those that can be controlled. Keeping careful records can help you identify the specific triggers of your bowel problems and how you react to them. This can help take some of the unpredictability out of your symptoms and pave the way for taking more control of them.

- *Monitoring helps you evaluate your progress.* It probably took a long time for you to get to this point; it will take some time to master your new skills. You may not see the full benefit of our program for a month or so. Careful records will help you figure out which strategy works best for which symptom in which situation. Your progress can be judged against the severity of symptoms you experience early on.

- *Monitoring keeps you motivated.* Especially in the beginning, keeping records helps you keep your eye on the goal until you start to see clear improvements in your ability to manage IBS. Having those records to look back on later will mean you'll be more likely to keep practicing the techniques that helped you the most. Keeping good records is also a nice way to give yourself credit for what you accomplish.

- *Monitoring helps you learn new skills.* Keeping good records will help you convert the knowledge you've learned about IBS into concrete new skills for managing symptoms and incorporating them into everyday life.

- *Monitoring helps you think objectively.* None of us knows everything about our bowel symptoms and our reactions to them. Even people who may have kept records in the past are surprised by how much more there is to learn about how symptoms unfold. Monitoring creates a little distance between you and your symptoms so that you can see the big picture more clearly. Making changes in behavior is a lot easier when you're able to step back and think objectively about the problems you want to change.

Now It's Your Turn

The first thing you need to do is track your symptoms and your stressful situations.

Tracking symptoms Each day, record your symptoms in the Daily IBS Diary, using the form on page 238 (see sample on page 73). You want to keep track of your symptoms and how severe they are. Write a number from 0 (none) to 8 (very severe) that describes the severity of each symptom. The diary also includes a space where you can record what medications you use to relieve your symptoms.

Tracking stress Once you track your symptoms, you want to see how they may relate to what's going on in your life. To do so, use the Daily Stress Worksheet on page 239 (see sample on pages 74-75). The worksheet includes space to write down details about stressful situations, what you were thinking while it happened, any reactions you had, and what you did to handle the situation. Carrying a copy of the worksheet will make it easier to keep up-to-date records. As soon as you notice an increase in your tension levels, log the situation and your reactions on the worksheet.

Column 1: Note the date of the event.

Column 2: Briefly describe the event or situation, where it took place, and who was there. Be specific without evaluating what the event meant to you.

Column 3: Describe what thoughts or images crossed your mind during or after the event.

Columns 4 and 5: Describe both your physical and emotional reactions to the event.

Column 6: Describe what you did to handle the situation.

It's important that you fill out the Daily Stress Worksheet completely for each situation you experience. Sometimes this will be easier than others. Just do your best to record all the information asked for on the form. Don't throw out your Daily Stress Worksheets—you'll use them for establishing patterns to bowel symptoms.

TO-DO LIST

- Use the IBS Diary to monitor your bowel symptoms every day.
- Use the Daily Stress Worksheet to track situations, physical sensations, thoughts, and behaviors over the next week.

Your Daily IBS Diary

IBS SEVERITY SCALE

0	1	2	3	4	5	6	7	8
NONE		**MILD**		**MODERATE**		**STRONG**		**SEVERE**

For each day, rate how much of a problem each symptom is using the 0-8 severity scale.

Date	Day	Pain or Discomfort	Diarrhea	Constipation	Sudden Urges	Bloating	Medication (type/amount)
Week #							
	Mon	2	3	0	1	0	Loperamide capsule 2mg 2x today
	Tue	6	7	0	3	5	Loperamide capsule 2mg 2x today
	Wed	7	8	0	6	6	
	Thu	6	5	0	3	3	
	Fri	1	1	0	2	0	
	Sat	0	0	0	0	0	
	Sun	2	2	0	1	4	
Week #							
	Mon						
	Tue						
	Wed						
	Thu						
	Fri						
	Sat						
	Sun						
Week #							
	Mon						
	Tue						
	Wed						
	Thu						
	Fri						
	Sat						
	Sun						

Daily Stress Worksheet

Date	What was the event?	What thoughts or images crossed your mind during and after the event?
12/04/06	Have work to prepare for presentation tomorrow	• I worry I won't do a good job. • I worry I won't be prepared. • I will not look prepared in front of audience coordinators. • I worry I'll stumble over my words. • I wish it could be canceled.
12/09/06	Traffic backed up on the 290 on way home	Head filled with a ticker tape of things I've got to do before tomorrow but can't because of this stupid traffic.
12/21/06	Argument with husband at breakfast	• I'll never make it to work on time thanks to him. • My supervisor will be on my case for sure. • My whole day is shot.
01/09/07	First date w/guy I really like	• What if I need to use the bathroom? • Worry he'll think I'm weird and never ask me out again.

What were your physical sensations while it was happening?	What were your feelings while it was happening?	What did you do to handle your feelings, thoughts, or bodily sensations?
Diarrhea, bloating, belly ached as I thought about presentation	• Worried • Nervous • Self-pity	Buried myself in office and studied my behind off
Tense shoulders and forehead	• Overwhelmed • Rushed • Pressure	Just listened to radio and watched traffic creep along
Belly pain, urge to go, bloating	• Frustrated • On edge • Tension • Impatience	Snarky, argumentative, slammed side door when leaving house, accidentally ran over sprinkler (broke it) when backing out of driveway
Tense, stomach in knot, diarrhea	• Keyed up • Worried • Stressed out!	Picked up the phone to cancel and tell him my boss called me in to work

STEP 2

TAKING CONTROL OF YOUR BODY WITH RELAXATION SKILLS

Sarah hated to speak in front of an audience. Whenever she knew she had to present a workshop to her staff, it seemed her anxiety levels increased and triggered IBS symptoms. Until she tracked her symptoms, she didn't realize that when she reached the podium, her muscles would tense, her heartbeat quickened, her stomach would tighten into a knot, and her breathing became shallow, rapid, and from her chest. The more she breathed like this, the tenser she got and the more she thought about tripping over her words and embarrassing herself. It didn't help knowing that, no matter how inconvenient, she would soon feel an urge to rush to the bathroom.

As Sarah eventually discovered, feeling tense and stressed directly affects the way you breathe. But once you're able to learn how to take command of your breathing, you're much more likely to feel calm, relaxed, and in control. Because the goal of this program is to manage IBS symptoms by getting a handle on stress, the very first strategy you'll want to learn is how to breathe in a relaxed way.

In this chapter, you'll learn how to handle stress by taking control of your body—learning specific relaxation skills. The key to doing this is to first learn a relaxed way to breathe; once you've mastered that, you'll learn strategies for how to relax your muscles. You will receive specific suggestions and ideas about how relaxing can help you lessen your IBS symptoms. Relaxing will help you take more control over your body, and this will make you feel more confident about facing and overcoming life's challenges.

It may seem kind of silly to discover you're going to need to learn how to relax your breathing. After all, infants don't need breathing lessons! But that's because their breathing patterns are healthy. The next time you see a little baby taking a nap, check out her tummy as she sleeps. It rises with each breath in, and falls with each breath out. This pattern is called *diaphragmatic breathing*, because it relies on a dome-shaped muscle beneath the ribs called the diaphragm. When you breathe in, the diaphragm moves down and the lungs expand with air, drawing in oxygen. As you breathe out, the diaphragm moves up, and the lungs contract, expelling air.

Slow, deep breathing like this is very good for you, lowering your blood pressure and heart rate, increasing the supply of blood and oxygen to the heart and brain, and resetting the balance of brain and body. These physical changes in turn produce a variety of positive psychological effects such as reduced worry and anxiety, as well as improvements in your emotional well-being. During diaphragmatic breathing, each breath is smooth, even, and rhythmic. Diaphragmatic breathing eases the intake of oxygen and the elimination of carbon dioxide (one of the body's waste products) with the least amount of effort.

If you always breathe like a baby, you probably could skip this part of the book. The problem is that as you age, you develop some bad habits. You rely on your chest instead of your diaphragm to fill your lungs with air. This is called *chest breathing*, and it stimulates a network of nerves that controls your heart, stomach, and intestines. An important job of this part of the nervous system is to regulate digestion and the muscle contractions that eliminate solid waste. So when you breathe from your chest, it activates the parts of your nervous system that produce many uncomfortable sensations experienced during periods of stress. Chest breathing also supplies the muscles with more oxygen to fuel the cells in the body, preparing you to fight or flee.

When psychological stress activates the fight-or-flight response, problems arise: Because you aren't fleeing or fighting, there's no outlet for the surge of physical tension, so activating the fight-or-flight response during a stressful situation is a bit like pressing one foot on the accelerator and the other on the brake at the same time. Your body, like your car, revs up. Revving up your body like this can disrupt the delicate balance between oxygen and carbon dioxide that your body needs to stay on an even keel.

Chest breathing also makes it hard to draw air into the lowest part of the lungs, where there's a concentration of small blood vessels that carry oxygen to the cells. With these blood vessels on the sidelines, chest breathing can make you feel tense and out of breath.

Diaphragmatic breathing, on the other hand, activates the part of the nervous system that puts a brake on the fight-or-flight response. It's impossible to be physically relaxed and stressed at the same time, so that by controlling your breathing patterns you override the physical part of stress that can aggravate bowel symptoms. With diaphragmatic breathing, there's a good mix of oxygen coming into the lungs and carbon dioxide coming out, and the fight-or-flight system comes to a screeching halt. Diaphragmatic breathing also releases the body's own painkillers (called endorphins), so you'll feel more comfortable.

Okay, ready to start learning how to breathe your way to stress-proof living?

CONTROLLED BREATHING STEP BY STEP

Step 1: Find a quiet, comfortable place free from distraction. Close your eyes so you won't be distracted. Practice this exercise either sitting in a comfortable chair or lying down.

Step 2: Place one hand on your belly above your belly button and the other hand on your chest. Don't try to change your breathing—just observe how you breathe. Notice which hand rises the most as you inhale. If you're using your diaphragm, your belly will push out and lift your bottom hand during the inhalation phase, while your top hand rests rock still on your chest (it's okay to look fat!). If your belly doesn't move or moves less than your chest, then you're breathing from your chest and your top hand will rise with each breath.

Step 3: Draw a normal amount of air deep into the bottom of your lungs.

Every time you breathe in this way, your abdomen expands. When you breathe out, the abdomen is sucked back in. You can relax your breathing by imagining that you're blowing up and deflating a large balloon inside your belly.

If You're Having Trouble Keeping Your Chest Still, Try This

- Breathe out all the air from your lungs. Draining air creates a vacuum that you'll find easy to fill by inhaling from your diaphragm.

- Alternatively, think about what it feels like to perform everyday tasks (such as yawning or having a bowel movement) that rely heavily on abdominal muscles.

Step 4: Inhale slowly and deeply, drawing air deeply into your lungs—just enough to inflate your abdomen. There's no need to take huge, fast gulps of air. Some people prefer to breathe in through their nose and breathe out through their mouth. Don't let the air out all at once after you breathe in; allow the air to flow evenly as you breathe in and out. You can control the amount of air you breathe out by gently pursing your lips as if you were blowing through a straw.

Step 5: To keep your breathing at a good, comfortable pace, count *one* to yourself as you breathe in. As you breathe out, picture the word *relax* or any focus words (such as *let go*) or image that conveys a calm, relaxed state as you relax. Count *two* when you breathe in and picture your focus word when you breathe out. Count up to 10 and then go back to the beginning and count again.

Step 6: Your only concern during the exercise is locking your attention on counting and monitoring the relaxed sensation as you exhale and repeat your focus word. If your attention drifts, just ease it back to the task at hand. With practice, you'll be able to count and imagine the focus word without any other thoughts popping into your head.

BREATHE YOUR WAY TO RELAXATION

Now that you've learned how to breathe correctly from your diaphragm, you can start practicing this breathing exercise. Do this exercise either sitting in a comfortable chair or lying down.

1. Find a comfortable, quiet location free of interruptions.

2. Gently close your eyes so you're not distracted.

3. Count *one* as you breathe in, and say *relax* as you breathe out. With each exhalation, part your lips and gently exhale as if you were trying to flicker the flame of a candle without extinguishing it, or blow across a spoonful of soup without spilling a drop.

4. As you breathe in, your belly should push out; as you breathe out, draw your belly in. Keep your chest still throughout.

5. Focus your attention on the number or relaxing word without letting other thoughts cross your mind.

6. Maintain a comfortable rate of breathing that is even and smooth.

7. Count up to 10 and repeat.

8. Practice two to three times daily for at least 10 minutes.

MUSCLE RELAXATION TRAINING

Now that you've got your breathing under control, it's time to move on to other tools for easing physical tension. And of course, you know that IBS symptoms can be aggravated by physical tension. People with IBS are often so busy getting things done and tending to everyone else's needs that they aren't aware of how much tension builds up inside them during the day. The only time they notice body tension is when it triggers bowel symptoms.

It's much easier to *prevent* tension than to try to *reduce* it once it occurs. The good news for people with IBS is that it's not hard to prevent or reduce physical tension by learning muscle relaxation exercises. In fact, studies have shown that IBS treatments featuring relaxation training are effective in decreasing IBS symptoms.

Now, you may be saying to yourself: "Relaxation exercises aren't going to work for me because I relax every day and I still have bowel problems!" If that's true for you, it's probably because what you consider "relaxation" is different from the physical relaxation designed to reduce IBS symptoms. People often think of relaxing as doing something they enjoy, such as gardening or watching a favorite TV program. Some of us even consider vigorous activities such as swimming or tennis as relaxation. Although these activities often reduce *mental* tension, they don't cause the *physical* changes that come with physical relaxation—and it's these physical changes that help control IBS.

The Relaxation Response

Physical relaxation refers to a process that produces a set of physical changes called the *relaxation response*. When you're physically relaxed, fewer nerve impulses travel from your muscles to your brain, dampening activity in the brain where pain and other gut sensations are registered. As your brain and body quiet down, you need less oxygen. Your breathing becomes deeper and slower. Your heart rate slows. The amount of blood pumped with each heartbeat decreases, lowering your blood pressure. The blood vessels relax and open. The production of hormones and chemicals falls. In effect, learning physical relaxation skills puts the emergency brake on your stress-triggered fight-or-flight response. Overall, the relaxation response stabilizes your body. That's why in the second half of this chapter, you're going to learn exactly how to relax your muscles.

Make Time to Relax

The first thing you want to do is think carefully about where and when to practice the relaxation skills that you're going to learn. You want to carve out 10 minutes of uninterrupted time twice each day. In today's busy world, taking time for yourself is hard! You may find that it's easier to pay attention to the needs of others before you worry about yourself. That's why you must give priority to your relaxation exercises, particularly in the beginning of this program when you're developing your new skills. If you find excuses for not practicing—such as being too busy—then that's probably a sign that you're most in need of this lesson!

If you're having a hard time practicing regularly, try to schedule a fixed time for relaxation every day, such as after dinner, right after you wake up in the morning, the 10 minutes after the kids are in bed, or before going to sleep. While once a day is the bare minimum to really learn the relaxation techniques, it will help if you can devote two or three periods each day to practicing in a place free of distractions. You may have to ask for help from your partner or family members. You may need to explain why it's important for you to do the exercises.

Of course, once you've learned how to relax, the process will take less and less time. In a few weeks, you'll find you're able to relax in just a minute or two. You'll find that you can do other, simpler relaxation exercises as you go about your day. For example, in the time it takes you to ride the elevator at your office, you can relax yourself with one deep breathing cycle. You can even do these quick exercises while riding in a car or watching television.

Find the Right Setting

Once you've figured out when you plan to do the exercises, you'll need to find a good place to practice.

- Look for a private place where you won't be disturbed, such as a bedroom, your office—even a bathroom. You will have plenty of opportunity to practice relaxation skills in the real world, but at this point your priority is to learn the relaxation skills in a quiet, controlled setting with minimal distraction.

- Pick a place without too many lights or distracting sounds. If possible, close the curtains and dim the lights.
- It's important that you're not interrupted. Turn off the answering machine. Tell family members to leave you alone while you practice. Hang a "Do Not Disturb" sign outside the door. Do whatever is necessary to guarantee you'll be left alone for the entire exercise period.
- Treat the relaxation exercises as you would any other self-care activity, such as going to the bathroom or brushing your teeth. Odds are you wouldn't say to yourself: "I don't have time to brush my teeth today. I can do it tomorrow or the next day when I have less to do. I'm just too busy."
- Choose a comfortable reclining chair or a couch that supports your head—as long as your body is comfortable and well supported.
- You want to be as comfortable as possible during your relaxation exercises. Wear loose-fitting clothing, take off your glasses, shoes, and watch. Make sure to cool off and calm down before beginning.
- Notice the points where your back and buttocks touch the chair, the floor, or the bed. Just let the chair, floor, or bed support those points.

Now you're ready to start learning how to relax.

Get into the Right Frame of Mind

Learning to relax your muscles is as much a mental exercise as it is a physical skill, and the most important thing is to learn how to be mentally calm while you relax. Here are some simple tips for helping you to become physically and mentally calm while practicing the exercises:

- *Get comfortable.* Let your limbs rest lightly on the recliner, bed, or couch. No part of your body should be touching any other part. Let your lips and teeth be slightly parted.

- *Let your eyes close when relaxing.* This will help you to concentrate on the exercises instead of what's going on around you.

- *Don't rush through the exercises.* Remember, the goal is not to rush—the goal is to learn ways to lessen physical tension.

- *Maintain a passive attitude.* Let yourself relax without trying too hard. Because relaxation is a skill you're capable of learning, there's no need to worry about how you're doing or whether you're doing it right. If your mind wanders during relaxation practice, don't be discouraged. Losing focus is normal at first. If you notice that thoughts pop into your mind, just let them float by, and gently refocus your attention on the relaxation exercise. Concentration is a skill that improves with practice.

- *After completing the exercise, pay attention to the sense of relaxation you created.* As you become more relaxed, take stock of the mental and physical changes you've noticed. Take a "mental snapshot" of what relaxation feels like. With daily practice, you'll be able to trigger it again quickly when you need it during your daily activities.

- *When you finish your relaxation, don't stand up quickly and rush off.* Because relaxation can lower your heart rate and blood pressure, give yourself time to become alert gradually before getting up. Sit up for a few moments. Enjoy the sensations of relaxation you created. Leave a little extra time at the end of your session for this purpose. Never set an alarm clock to signal the end of your relaxation session.

PROGRESSIVE MUSCLE RELAXATION

Okay, now you're ready to take the first step in learning how to relax your body and your mind. If you're like most people who need to relax, you'll probably get halfway through this exercise and start wondering how you're doing, whether you're relaxing enough, or whether it's taking too long. Just let go of those thoughts! Relaxation is the kind of thing where the more you try to relax, the less likely you are be to succeed. The best approach is to intend to relax but to be a bit detached about how you are doing. Because relaxation is a skill everyone can learn with a bit of patience and practice, you know that eventually you'll master it!

The first thing you're going to want to focus on is how to relax your muscles. Most people never really understand how tense and tight their muscles can get in the course of a day, because most of us are pretty much out of touch with our bodies. And while we think that everyone *should* know how to relax, in fact it's a skill, just like learning how to ride a bike or drive a car.

Progressive muscle relaxation is a clinically proven self-management exercise that involves tensing and then relaxing individual muscle groups. This is an important skill to learn for a couple of reasons. By tensing the muscles *before* you relax, you're actually making it easier to achieve muscle relaxation afterward. Think of muscle relaxation as sort of like a pendulum. If you want the pendulum to swing in a particular direction, then you first have to pull it back in the opposite direction and then let go. Relaxing your muscles works on the same principle. By tensing your muscles, you create momentum that allows you to deepen muscle relaxation. The tensing procedure also helps you take a clear mental snapshot of what muscles feel like when they are tense, so you can detect tension once it appears later, and control it before it builds up and becomes a problem. Many times, people realize they are tense only when that tension reaches significant levels. If you can detect tension earlier, then you can do something about it before it gets out of control.

Read the following set of instructions to learn how to tense each muscle group. But remember: While you're tensing one set of muscles, the rest of your body must be relaxed. The tendency at the beginning is to allow the muscles in your entire body to tense up at the same time, but that's not what you're after here. It can take some practice to be able to isolate and relax a muscle.

1. Lie down, or sit in a comfortable chair with your arms and hands supported. Be sure to loosen any tight clothing. Close your eyes so you're not easily distracted, and breathe evenly, quietly, and slowly.

2. Focus on the muscles of your left hand and left lower arm. Tense these muscles by making a tight fist with your hands, tensing each muscle group enough to feel tightness without pain or discomfort. Pay attention as the tension spreads from your fingers and hand, over the knuckles, across the wrist, and through the lower arm. Study the tension in your arm and hand, and then relax those muscles. As your muscles relax, notice how they feel now compared to what they felt like when they were tense. Allow your hand and arm to settle into your lap, feeling relaxed warm, and loose.

3. Next, focus on the muscles of the left biceps. You'll want to tense these bicep muscles by pushing your elbow down against the arm (or seat) of a chair. Feel the tightness of just the biceps. Study the tension and hold it for 10 seconds. Now, "turn off" the tension and relax. Study the contrast between the tension and relaxation.

4. Repeat steps 2 and 3 for the right hand and biceps.

5. Now focus on the muscles of the face. Lift your eyebrows as high as possible and wrinkle your forehead. Concentrate on the tension you created across your forehead. (There's no need to overdo it when you tense the muscles. You don't want to tense them so much that you strain your muscles.) Hold the tension for about 10 seconds. Study it. Concentrate on the tension and then relax the muscles. Pay attention to the difference between the tension and the pleasant sense of relax-

ation in your muscles as they smooth out, unwind, and relax more deeply. Enjoy the contrast between the tension and relaxation. For the next 30 seconds or so, enjoy the relaxation you created before moving to the next step.

6. Squint your eyes (be careful if you wear contact lenses) and wrinkle your nose so that you feel tension in your jaws and upper cheeks. Hold the tension. Study how hard and tense the muscles feel. Concentrate on the tension. Take a mental snapshot of what the tension feels like. Now relax, releasing the tension, focusing on the pleasant sense of relaxation flowing into your muscles. Study the difference between the tension and the relaxation you created. Let your muscles relax further and further, and enjoy what that feels like.

7. Bite your teeth and clench your jaw while pulling back the corners of your mouth as if you were making an exaggerated grin. Notice the tension in your jaw, and the whole facial area. Hold the tension you created. Study it. Concentrate on the tension. Now let go and relax, letting your lips part and jaw loosen. Again, notice the difference between the tension and relaxation.

8. Tense your neck muscles by pulling your chin toward your chest while pressing the back of your head on the back of the chair or bed. Concentrate on the tension in the back of your neck and base of your head. Study the tension. Concentrate on the tightness for about 10 seconds or so. Turn off the tension, relaxing the neck muscles and letting your head return to a comfortable position. Pay attention to the difference between the tension and the relaxation.

9. Now focus on the muscles of the shoulders. Raise your shoulders together so that they nearly touch the bottom of your ears. See how this increases tension in your shoulders, upper back, and neck? Study the tightness, and hold it for 5 seconds. Now relax. As if you were

snipping a string connecting your shoulder to your ears, let your shoulders drop further and further to a resting position. Just keep letting go of the muscles in your shoulders until relaxation spreads deep into the shoulders and back muscles. Take a mental snapshot of what the muscle relaxation feels like.

10. Take a deep breath and hold the air long enough to tighten the muscles in your stomach. Hold the tension. Notice the tension as your abdomen hardens. Now relax, let go of the tension, and notice the contrast between the tension and relaxation. Just let the muscles loosen, relax, smooth out.

11. Moving on to the legs and feet, stretch out your right leg so it is straight and then flex your toes toward your head. Feel the tension in your thigh. Concentrate on it. Study it. Now relax your foot and leg. Compare the tension and relaxation you created.

12. Extend your left leg and flex the toes back toward your head. Study the tension in your left leg. Concentrate on it. Study it. And now relax. Compare the tension and relaxation you created.

As you progress through the tension-relaxation cycles, your whole body will feel more and more relaxed. Notice the difference between the tension and relaxation you create. Just release the tension, focusing on the muscles as they relax. At this point, you should scan your body for any tension in your muscles. If you find any areas of tension, just concentrate on those muscles, release the tension, and the relaxation will increase.

Notice what it feels like as the muscles become more and more relaxed. Enjoy the feeling of deep relaxation as the muscles go on relaxing more and more completely. There is nothing for you to do but to focus your attention on the very pleasant sensation of deep relaxation flowing through your muscles. When you've relaxed your entire body, enjoy the feeling of physical relaxation you created. Your body will settle comfortably into the chair or bed. All your muscles will feel looser and more deeply relaxed.

Once you learn to use progressive muscle relaxation to achieve deep relaxation, the next step is to apply this skill to your everyday life whenever tension crops up. You can learn this skill by shortening the exercise so you relax faster. To do this, you can reduce the number of muscle groups you relax. For example, you can tense the muscles of your right or left hand, forearm, and upper arm all at once by making a tight fist of your hand and raising your hand toward your shoulder. Instead of tensing individual muscle groups in your face, tense the muscles in your forehead, upper cheeks, lower face, and jaw, all at once. Just release the tension, allowing the relaxation to spread and enjoy the feelings in the muscles as they spread out, loosen, and relax more deeply and completely.

CUE-CONTROLLED RELAXATION

A more advanced exercise for relaxing more quickly is called *cue-controlled relaxation*. With this exercise, you can reduce tension without going through the tension relaxation cycles of progressive muscle relaxation. Cue-controlled relaxation involves pairing a cue word or phrase with relaxation exercise. It's called cue-controlled relaxation because the cue phrase serves as a cue for the relaxation response.

Read over the following exercise a couple of times to familiarize yourself with cue-controlled relaxation. Then begin. With practice and patience, you'll soon find that this is a handy, portable relaxation exercise that you can use during the day whenever you begin to feel tense and uneasy.

1. Sit or lie down in a comfortable position.

2. Close your eyes. Place your hands loosely in your lap.

3. Take slow, even, deep breaths from the diaphragm, not the chest. Make sure you breathe in at a slow, unhurried, and regular pace. Hold your breath for a count of one and exhale for a count of four.

Focus on the breaths you take. Feel the cool air pass through your nostrils on the inhalation and the warm air pass through your lips when you breathe out.

4. As you pay attention to your breathing, silently repeat the phrase: *I am relaxed.* When you inhale, say *I am*, and as you exhale, silently repeat the word *relaxed.* As you do this, focus on the muscles across your forehead, picturing the tension leaving your body with every exhalation.

5. As your forehead muscles relax, move down to the facial area, mentally repeating the phrase *I am relaxed.*

6. Relax the eye muscles. As these muscles relax, move on to the mouth area. Relax.

7. Now focus your concentration on the area around your back and neck, and relax. This is an area where stress can really build up, so take your time here. Don't move on until you really feel the muscles of the back of your neck loosen up and relax.

8. Next, move to the muscles at the back of your shoulders.

9. Now focus on the muscles of your chest and arms, and relax.

10. Move on to the rest of your body, muscle group by muscle group, until you reach your feet.

11. When you've gotten to the muscles of your feet, just sit a few minutes and enjoy the feeling of total muscle relaxation. Slowly open your eyes, and after some time, you may get up.

Most people find this exercise to be a nice way of relaxing the body when they feel stressed, anxious, or tense. Pay attention for signs of muscle tension during the day—stiffness in your back, tightness in your neck, knots in your stomach, clenched teeth, raised shoulders. These sensations can cue you to begin this relaxation exercise. Say you are in the middle of a difficult work assignment and you notice that your jaws and shoulders feel stiff and tense. This can cue you to use the relaxation exercise described here. To get the most out of this exercise, you may want to scan your body two or three times a day for signs of tension.

Pick a regular time to use this exercise—when you get in to your office and check your messages first thing in the morning, when you return from lunch, take a break from some task, or when you feel that "mid-afternoon slump" around 3 or 4 P.M. Try this technique in different situations and postures such as standing, sitting, or walking.

As you practice these exercises, don't worry if you notice some unusual sensations, such as a tingling or a heavy feeling. Those are normal responses caused by physical relaxation of the muscles. In fact, these sensations are a sure sign that you're getting control of your body!

RELAXATION COUNTDOWN

After you've practiced breathing or progressive muscle relaxation methods, you may want to learn a countdown procedure as a way of deepening the sensation of muscle relaxation you create. With this technique, you'll be able to relax in situations that cause tension—even in the middle of a busy day—giving you lots more control over how your body reacts to stress. This exercise is helpful when you find yourself getting tense at work or at home. Rather than allowing stress to build up, use the first signs of tension, distressing thoughts, or anxiety as a cue to relax.

1. Sit or lie down and close your eyes.

2. Release muscle tension using one of the two methods described.

3. Once all your muscles are totally relaxed, begin counting backward slowly, from five to one.

4. As you mentally say the number five, imagine yourself either walking down stairs, descending an escalator, or floating in a balloon, feeling more deeply relaxed. With each number, you feel yourself becoming

more and more deeply relaxed.

5. As you count, keep imagining yourself descending into a state of deeper and deeper relaxation.

6. After every couple of numbers, you will find yourself becoming more and more deeply relaxed until you reach one, when you will feel completely relaxed. Don't rush the countdown. Wait to go to the next number until you're really relaxing. As you count down, you will feel yourself becoming more deeply relaxed.

7. Now it's time to move out of the relaxation period, counting from five to one. On the count of four, you can move your legs and feet. On the count of three, you can move your arms and hands. On the count of two, you can move your head and neck. On the count of one, gently open your eyes and you'll feel completely relaxed.

VISUALIZATION

As your body relaxes, so does your brain. The opposite is also true—as your mind becomes more relaxed, your body relaxes. One way to deepen your feelings of relaxation is through visualization exercises. Many athletes and dancers incorporate the visualization exercises described here to give them a competitive edge for peak performance. When you do a visualization relaxation exercise, you're basically creating a word, phrase, or mental image in your "mind's eye." The idea behind visualizaton was stated by Henry Ford: "If you think you can or you think you can't, you're usually right."

Athletes use visualization to rehearse their moves before performing them. World-class skiers imagine themselves negotiating every inch of a hairpin turn on a ski slope, hockey players picture where in the net they want to shoot a puck, and gymnasts visualize each step of their routine before actually performing each maneuver. This technique is as relevant to medical patients wanting more control of their bodies as it is to athletes. Because the body does not distinguish between an event that occurs in the here and now and one that is imagined, what we visualize can affect our body as much as a real experience.

One key to effective visualization is calling to mind a nice, safe, pleasant place. The more clearly you can bring this place to mind, the deeper your relaxation experience. To do this, try to imagine details, including sounds, sights, textures, and smells. Many people find lying on a beach a relaxing scene that they can easily incorporate into their relaxation exercises. However, don't just recall a simple memory of the ocean. Get all your senses involved to create what an ocean scene is really like. Smell the salty spray of ocean mist in the air and feel the occasional cool breeze grazing your cheeks. Hear the playful squawk of the seagulls, the crash of waves rolling rhythmically onto the shore. Feel the warmth of the sun on your head, your back, your legs, and the fleecy blanket you're lying on, warmed by the soft white sand. Smell the hot dogs grilling over the fire. Picture the white, soft, puffy clouds floating against the deep blue sky. Let all of your senses transport you to this image.

Now sit or lie down, and close your eyes and follow the visualization steps below.

1. Choose a place you find relaxing, calm, and peaceful—a deserted beach, a mountaintop, the woods, a garden, nature trail, or a pasture by a brook. You can either pick a place that you have been to or just visualize a place you've always wanted to visit to escape the pressures of daily life. If you have trouble concentrating on your image, use physical cues from your immediate surrounding to jump-start your visualization skills. Flowers in the room, for example, may help you recall the pleasant, peaceful surroundings of a walk through a garden.

2. Close your eyes and focus vividly on the image you have selected. As

you imagine details of your relaxing scene, allow yourself as much comfort or pleasure as you can. Just let go. There's nothing to do and nowhere to go, so you might as well enjoy and relax. Don't force a particular image to stay in your mind. Let your mind go naturally to your relaxing place. It's okay to wander within your image. Let yourself enjoy the pleasant moment for as long as you want. You may find that it's not so bad to feel relaxed and comfortable.

3. When you feel you're finished with the relaxation and want to return to a normal state of alertness, just count backward from five to one. With each number you will feel more alert and awake. When you get to one, your eyes will open and you will be awake, refreshed, and comfortable.

Make Your Own Relaxation Tape

If you have trouble remembering the steps in the muscle relaxation exercises, you may want to simply make your own relaxation tape by recording the steps and then playing it back during your practice periods. Remember to give yourself enough time between steps. By recording your own tape, you can tailor an exercise that works for you. If you're making a tape of progressive muscle relaxation exercise, tense each muscle group for about 5 seconds before relaxing them for 10 to 15 seconds. Give yourself 20 to 30 seconds to concentrate on the pleasurable relaxation sensation before proceeding to the next muscle group. If you're recording breathing exercises, try to shoot for about 10 breaths per minute. That works out to about 3 seconds per inhalation and 3 seconds per exhalation. The entire relaxation exercise should last no more than 15 to 20 minutes.

When you're ready to record, begin reading at a slow, regular pace, using a relaxed voice. Don't rush to complete the recording. Relaxation can't be hurried—just let it happen, and it will. A relaxation tape can help you learn basic skills, but you don't want to rely on the tape, or else it will be hard to apply relaxation skills to real-life situations.

TRACK YOUR PROGRESS

Keeping a record before and after each relaxation session is a good way to see the progress you're making. You can use the Relaxation Training Worksheet on page 240 (see a sample of a completed worksheet on the next page). In order to chart your progress, you want to assign a number to how relaxed you were before and after the session.

Most people aren't used to assigning numbers to express the amount of relaxation they're feeling, but it's easy to do. The relaxation scale runs from 0 to 100, with 0 meaning no relaxation at all and 100 meaning the highest level of relaxation imaginable; 25 would be a small amount of relaxation, while 75 would indicate a high level of relaxation.

Use the same scale to record how well you concentrated during the relaxation exercises. A score of 0 means that your concentration is weak and you were easily distracted, while a score of 100 means that you were able to keep focused on relaxation exercises and weren't thinking about anything else. A score of 50 means that your concentration drifted but was sometimes focused. Your goal by the end of next week is to achieve levels of relaxation and concentration of at least 60.

TO-DO LIST

- Practice the relaxation exercises on a daily basis. To get the most out of the exercises, practice twice a day for 10 minutes at a time. If you can't practice twice a day, once is okay, but it may lengthen the time it takes for you to feel more relaxed in general. If you don't practice regularly, you probably won't get the benefits of the exercises.
- Record each practice session on the Relaxation Training Worksheet.
- Continue to use the worksheets to track the situations, thoughts, reactions, and bowel problems you experience over the next week.

Relaxation Training Worksheet

0	10	20	30	40	50	60	70	80	90	100
None		**Mild**		**Moderate**			**Strong**		**Extreme**	

Rate your relaxation and concentration using the above scale each time you practice.
In the last column, jot down anything that happens while you practiced.

Date	Practice Session	Relaxation at end of practice session	Concentration during practice session	Comments
5/1/07	First	60	70	Felt good. A lot easier than I
	Second	60	60	thought. Focus a little off today
5/2/07	First	70	60	Concentration better,
	Second	70	70	so relaxing
5/3/07	First	No time	No time	Was really overwhelmed today
	Second	70	80	Only practiced 1 time
5/4/07	First	70	70	Racing thoughts, weaker
	Second	60	50	reaction
5/5/07	First	60	60	Hard to breathe out with
	Second	50	60	stomach in
5/6/07	First	70	80	Really helped with work
	Second	80	80	pressure
5/7/07	First	70	70	Feel like I'm improving!
	Second	80	70	
5/8/07	First	70	60	
	Second	70	60	
5/9/07	First	60	60	Disrupted by two phone calls
	Second	60	50	
5/10/07	First	70	70	Concentration better then
	Second	80	80	yesterday. Felt really good!
5/11/07	First	70	50	Son interrupted me–never got
	Second	80	60	on track
5/12/07	First	80	70	Tension levels ↓, Relaxation ↑
	Second	80	80	
5/13/07	First	90	80	Proud of myself!
	Second			

STEP 3

APPLYING RELAXATION SKILLS TO EVERYDAY LIFE

Paul is a hard-driving oil company executive who had been suffering with IBS for several years—and the more stressful his career became, the worse his symptoms got. That is, until he learned some relaxation techniques, which he practiced until he was able to quickly relax himself in a matter of minutes. When things got tense and worries would get the best of him, he'd close his office door, take a couple of minutes to sit back, close his eyes, breathe deeply, and let his muscles go limp. In less than half a minute he'd begin to feel calmer and less tense, better able to concentrate and more alert.

As Paul discovered, relaxation exercises can really help you get a handle on stress. Did you find the relaxation exercises described in the previous chapter to be helpful? Did your level of relaxation and concentration improve the more you practiced? Did you set aside enough time for the exercises?

Like any new skill, there are probably a few kinks to work out, but if you have practiced regularly, you've probably found that the exercises are already helping you relax and feel more in control of your body. That's an experience that's not familiar to many people with IBS, so pat yourself on the back if you were able to achieve at least a moderate level of relaxation.

Don't get discouraged if you initially struggle with the exercises—you should work at a pace that allows you to learn new skills. When you were first learning to drive a car, you may have forgotten to signal. Maybe you drove too slowly, or you had trouble parallel parking. Chances are you didn't give up and say "Forget it, I'm just going to take the bus from now on." With practice, you learned from your experiences, made adjustments, and plugged along. Your skills gradually improved until driving seemed automatic.

That's how it will be as you're learning relaxation skills. Because relaxation feels good, it's one health behavior you can enjoy learning.

It sure is a lot more fun than flossing your teeth! The enjoyment you get out of relaxation training will make it more likely you'll do it again.

MAKE RELAXATION WORK FOR YOU

Now it's time to learn how to solve problems you may be having with your relaxation exercises. If you had trouble focusing on the exercises, or if you were interrupted a lot, here are some ways to reduce disruptions:

- If you feel mildly lightheaded or dizzy as you practice breathing, you may have been taking in too much air. Slow down your breathing so that breathing in takes about four seconds and breathing out takes about six seconds.
- If you're interrupted while relaxing, continue and deal with the problem later. Even after an interruption you may still get some benefit from completing the exercises.
- Talk to people who might interrupt you and explain the importance of the exercises and the need for quiet. If you can, get others to try the exercises with you to help them understand.
- Remind family members or coworkers that you won't be available while you're relaxing.
- If the place where you're relaxing isn't quiet enough, find a new one. Relax in an out-of-the way room with a door, and don't hesitate to use a Do Not Disturb sign.
- Try to eliminate outside noise. If you can't, use a fan to help drown out distracting background sounds.
- If you're falling asleep while relaxing, you may be too tired to get the most out of the exercises. Try to get more sleep, and practice relaxation when you're more awake. You may want to change the place where you relax—for example, try moving from the bed to a chair.

During the early phase of relaxation training, you've been practicing in a quiet, comfortable place free of distractions. If you're feeling more

Solving Problems

The following questions may help you identify and work around any problems you've had with the relaxation exercises. Use this information to develop an action plan to improve your relaxation skills.

- What problems have you had while doing your relaxation exercises?
- What have you done to solve these problems?
- What, if anything, has worked?
- After reading this section, can you think of other things that may work to help you concentrate on your relaxation exercises?

comfortable using the exercises, the next step is to apply your skills to more everyday situations or when you first feel an increase in body tension coming on. This step will give you a portable tool for combating stress during your regular routine.

Over the next week, take a number of mini relaxation breaks during the day in a variety of settings:

- Sitting upright in a chair
- Sitting in a restaurant
- Typing on the computer
- Waiting in a checkout line
- Walking outside
- Standing in the living room
- Watching TV
- Sitting in a theater

Once you start to feel tense, use those stressful feelings as a cue to concentrate on slow, smooth, deep breathing. Count *1* while breathing in and think *relax* while breathing out deeply and evenly. Count up to 10 and back to 1. Breathe at a rate of about 8 to 12 breaths per minute. As you breathe slowly, let your tense muscles loosen and relax. You can deepen your physical relaxation by thinking of a pleasant scene—relaxing on a beach, taking a hike in the countryside, or picnicking in a pine forest. Whatever works for you.

You can practice your relaxation breaks any time you feel stress—not just when you're sitting at home in your easy chair. Try your techniques when you're trapped in traffic on your way to work or stuck in a long line at the bank. If you enjoy sports, try the technique right before swinging a golf club, diving off the high dive, or taking a basketball shot. Or try the techniques right before you walk out on stage to give a talk to that intimidating group of cardiologists at your next professional conference.

You'll be amazed at what a difference it makes if you can devote about two minutes several times a day to simple relaxation methods. You'll find that breathing more slowly and loosening your muscles can do your body and mind good. If you make a point of doing this, you'll decrease your stress level and reap a number of health benefits.

TO-DO LIST

- Continue to practice the relaxation exercises every day.
- Record each practice session on the Relaxation Training Worksheet. Continue to use the worksheet to track the situations, thoughts, reactions, and bowel problems you experience over the next week.
- Practice taking mini relaxation breaks throughout the week, in all kinds of situations.

STEP 4

OUTSMART IBS BY TRACKING YOUR THOUGHTS

Janet, 19, is a college student working her way through school at the information desk at the university library. Even though she has excellent grades, her gut acts up like clockwork at the end of the semester when she is under the gun to balance schoolwork and her job schedule. In addition to cramps and constipation, Janet has been bothered by gurgling noises coming from her stomach. Because she works in a place of particular quiet, she was really starting to get sensitive that other students would walk by and hear her stomach rumbling while they studied. It got so bad that every day on her way to work she'd anxiously wish that no one would approach her desk. "What if someone hears my stomach growl? What will they think of me?" Most days she arrived at work with a huge knot deep in her belly.

Janet's situation shows the powerful role thoughts have on your body reactions. In this chapter, you'll learn how you can start changing those thoughts in more constructive ways. In this step of the program an important goal will be to pay more attention to your thoughts over the next week and then learn how to control them. This will help you target the mental tension triggered by certain thoughts, interpretations, beliefs, and expectations.

This step is important, because scientists have learned that it's not an event itself, but how we *think* about that event that determines our reactions. In other words, that important board meeting itself isn't what makes you stressed, tense, or angry—it's your interpretation or belief *about* that board meeting that triggers uncomfortable reactions. You can change your reactions by changing the way you think about things. In addition, the way you think about things or events can directly affect your feelings, your behavior, and your physical responses.

The power of thoughts and beliefs to influence your reactions explains why two people can react very differently to the same event. This is why some people who get stuck in a traffic jam feel furious and restless, while others just take it in stride. All you need to do is to recognize that thinking influences your reactions—and you'll be on your way to improved digestive health.

As stress builds up, a person often begins to think negative thoughts. The comments you make to yourself (called *self-talk*) become more extreme as you overestimate both the likelihood of a problem happening, and how bad it will be. But the longer you hold on to extreme thoughts in stressful situations, the worse off you'll be. This is because these extreme thoughts don't fade away; negative self-talk directly affects how you feel and what you do, tipping the balance between health and illness, happiness and sadness, and confidence and vulnerability.

People who tend to automatically think the worst, or jump to conclusions, are more likely to respond more strongly to life's everyday hassles, and they are also more likely to have a harder time recovering. Researchers also have found that when you worry, chemical changes in the brain make physical pain more intense and less tolerable. Simply put, extreme thoughts lead to extreme reactions.

Luckily, you can learn how to tone down those extreme thoughts and help change your reactions that fuel the vicious cycle of IBS. The next steps in our program will tell you how. You'll learn ways to think more constructively, so that you can filter out stress *before* it has a chance to disrupt your digestive system. You can learn to recognize or change your reactions by changing your thinking patterns. To do this, we'll focus on the mental component of stress—worry.

GOOD vs. BAD WORRY

Worrying bothers almost everyone sometimes. Whenever you're facing problems, your mind is always trying to make sense of things. Worrying can help you solve problems and motivates you to perform at your best. But sometimes, worry can get the better of you. At its worst, worry can sabotage your goals, create emotional distress, and aggravate health problems.

Researchers who study the thinking style of people with IBS find that they can worry more than people without IBS. People with IBS typically experience two types of worrisome thoughts or bad worries:

- Worries about uncontrollable problems that have already occurred
- Worries about problems that haven't happened yet—and in most cases never will!

Because the things you worry about don't exist in the here and now, the only place they play out is in your head. At times, it's hard to turn worries off. Sometimes, they keep racing around in the back of the mind like a broken record.

Worry is a bit like cholesterol—just as there is good and bad cholesterol, there's good and bad worry. Worry that generates an action plan for solving an immediate problem is "good" worry. In good worry, you have a problem, you worry about it, you develop a plan of attack for fixing the problem, you take action, and solve the problem. End of story.

With bad worry, there's no immediate problem to solve. Your mind latches on to a problem that either already has happened or you think will someday happen—but can't be changed right now. Bad worry increases tension and can interfere with how the brain and gut interact with each other. Bad worry is often made up of phrases such as: "If only . . ." and "What if . . . "

- If only I had studied harder, I would have done better on the exam.
- If only I had left earlier, I wouldn't have been late for the meeting.
- If only I had taken my Mom to the doctor earlier, she wouldn't have gotten sick.

"If only" events have already occurred, but that doesn't stop your mind from trying to do something about the problem as a way of figuring out what went wrong and how to fix it. Have you ever found yourself dwelling on a past problem, regret, or disappointment? If so, you're not alone. When this happens, you forget that because the event has already occurred nothing can be done. But when your mind recalls the event, its natural tendency is to keep trying to solve the problem. Worry is a way of doing something about an event that didn't turn out the way you wanted.

On the other hand, "what if" thinking concerns predictions or expectations about the future. These thoughts focus on any number of possible threats, misfortunes, or catastrophes that might happen.

- What if my husband is late coming home from work . . . has he been in an accident?
- What if I can't find a bathroom and have an accident?
- What if I get lost while driving downtown?
- What if there is no one I know at the party?
- What if the electric company didn't get my check on time?
- What if I can't make the deadline on Friday?
- What if my stomach growls during the meeting with my boss?

There's no shortage of things to worry about. Life is constantly presenting us with a smorgasbord of worries. The worry smorgasbord can make you just as sick if you overdo it as the $4.95 All-You-Can-Eat Breakfast Buffet.

DO YOU WORRY TOO MUCH?

Most people worry if an unpleasant event happens and if it involves something or someone very important to them. Similarly, most of us worry if a likely bad event is coming our way. Your mind will try to figure out how to avoid a bad outcome if you have to drive in very bad weather, or if you're facing an important challenge at work where poor performance on your part is a real possibility.

If worrying is a natural way the mind responds to unpleasant events in the past or future, how can you decide how much worry is too much? There are two simple rules for determining "appropriate" worry.

Rule #1. If worrying about an immediate problem doesn't provide a quick solution, then simple worrying is not helpful and can be considered bad worry.

Keep in mind that worry is effective only if the impending event you're worrying about is really likely to happen and helps you come up with an action plan. If you feel abdominal pain and wonder: "What if it's stomach cancer?" this may prompt you to set up a doctor's appointment. Once the visit is scheduled, however, you've done all you can, and worry loses its helpfulness. Remember, there isn't any link between IBS and stomach cancer. So the chance that your symptoms mean you have cancer is very low—and persistent worrying about it doesn't make the situation any better. No amount of worrying will clarify the results of tests before the doctor has had a chance to review them. To continue worrying after the doctor rules out cancer is even less helpful.

Even for future bad events that are quite likely to happen, worry may not be useful and will simply cause more problems. This is what happens when you've done all the problem solving you can before the event, and there's nothing more you can do. Of course, it's natural for negative events in the past or future to attract your attention. But if you've done all you can reasonably do to prepare, to continue to worry merely causes more distress and interferes with the rest of your life.

But what about those times when you find yourself going over old problems that have already occurred, so that you're just rehashing past unpleasant events?

Rule #2. Unless thinking about a past mistake or regret helps you learn from that mistake, dwelling on the past won't help. Just let it go. It may not be desirable, but you really have no other choice.

Put these rules together, and what do they tell you? Unless worries help you solve an immediate problem or learn from one that just occurred, they're more trouble than they're worth. So let's see what practical tools you can learn to control worries before they get the best of you. Worrying may be natural, but it's not always helpful. That's why learning ways to control it can be useful. Many of your thoughts during stressful situations aren't always accurate—they're just guesses or predictions of what you expect will happen. Sometimes these predictions can be off base, and when this happens, these thoughts can take a toll on your mind and body. Once you realize that the way you size up events isn't necessarily accurate or useful, you're free to substitute more helpful ways of thinking.

First, look at what's behind these guesses. Research shows that during stress, people develop serious blind spots in their thinking that stop them from considering alternatives. For example, when the company's top sales-man gets an unusually lackluster sales report and thinks: "I'm just not up to this job," he's thinking the worst. When his officemate hears the rumor that her employer is considering layoffs, she says to herself: "If I lose my job, it would be terrible. There's no way I'd be able to get a new job before the bills start piling up. I'll have to move in with my parents and that would be the pits." She's dwelling on the worst-case scenario without factoring in her ability to cope with setbacks. This mental blind spot is called *blowing things out of proportion*. Just like the physical blind spots in a rearview mirror, these mental blind spots can prevent you from seeing things clearly and are physically hazardous if you're not aware of them.

You can eliminate mental blind spots by asking yourself whether you can look at the situation in a different way. Let's say your friend is worried about getting in front of a crowd and giving a presentation. You'd probably reassure her that everything will be fine and there's no sense in getting worked up over it. You're encouraging her to eliminate her mental blind spot—to let go of her worry. Your friend feels a lot better for the comforting advice you've given. But when the blind spot is your own, you may not always practice what you preach.

AUTOMATIC THINKING

One reason that thoughts are so hard to challenge is because they occur so automatically that you often aren't even aware of them. If you had to think about every detail of your life—opening a car door, walking, chewing a piece of toast—you'd be so bogged down in the details that there would be little time to do much else. Imagine how long it would take to talk yourself through each step of tying your shoelaces.

1. First you take one shoe, and lace it up with your shoelace.

2. To lace it up, crisscross your shoelace over and under the holes in your shoe.

3. When the ends of your shoelaces meet, take one end, lay the other down, then go over and under your laid-down end.

4. Take one end of your shoelace and make a loop.

5. Take the end of the lace and wrap it around the loop. By doing that, you make a smaller loop.

6. Put the middle of the shoelace you haven't looped through the small hole.

7. By putting your shoelace through the hole, you make another big loop.

8. Pull on the big loop very hard, this will make it tight.

9. Return to Step 1 and repeat with other shoe.

None of us ever really THINKS through all the steps as we tie our shoelaces. That's because ever since we were preschoolers, we've repeated these steps so many times they've become habits. Activities such as tying shoes, riding a bike, driving a car, and brushing your teeth in the morning are habits.

The way you think about things can become habitual, too. Worrying is an example of a mental habit that can become automatic and develop into a problem if you've done a lot of it in the past. As the habit of worrying gets stronger, you don't even notice the process anymore. Sometimes, your worries appear in code, composed of just a few "hot" words or a brief visual image. Typically, just a few words are all you need to trigger a cascade of physical and emotional reactions.

Imagine that your coworker tells you your boss wants to see you as soon as possible. Immediately your gut starts to cramp up and you're engulfed by a sense of dread. These reactions happen so fast it's hard to catch the exact thoughts that triggered your reactions. But remember— **situations alone don't trigger a reaction. It's your beliefs about what the situation means that make you respond the way you do.**

Automatic thoughts usually have several things in common:

• *No matter how irrational, automatic thoughts are accepted as facts.* For example, a woman whose son fails an exam worries that he won't get into his first-choice college. A woman assumes that her boyfriend has lost interest because he didn't return her email. Automatic thoughts are plausible; it often never occurs to us to question their accuracy. Because the content of our automatic thoughts seems plausible, they go unchallenged. But once you carefully examine the validity of your worries you realize that most automatic thoughts distort the truth, and while possible, are not very probable.

• *Automatic thoughts are extreme, and tend to "awfulize."* They predict catastrophe and misfortune, and make you expect the worst: A severe headache is a symptom of a brain tumor. A disappointing sales report triggers fears of job security. A woman who doesn't get a holiday card from her old roommate thinks the friend doesn't like her.

• *Automatic thoughts aren't useful because they're extreme and lead to strong emotional and physical reactions.* They don't help you solve problems right now. They force you to dwell on problems that have already occurred, or get you thinking about possible problems that aren't occurring right now.

• *Automatic thoughts are hard to turn off.* They seem to come and go with a will of their own—kind of like Internet pop-up ads of the mind.

• *Automatic thoughts are learned and habit-forming.* Ever since you were a kid, people have been telling you what to think, how to act, what to feel. You've been conditioned by family, friends, and the media to process information in a certain way. The way you think about events can become as much a habit as smoking, drinking a morning cup of coffee, brushing your teeth, using your seat belt, or saying hi to your coworkers every morning. Because automatic thoughts are learned, they can be unlearned, and replaced with more constructive ways of thinking that make you feel more comfortable in your own skin.

CONSTRUCTIVE THINKING

Once you make some simple changes to your thinking patterns, you can improve your ability to cope with stress and deal more effectively with various situations and experiences.

Changing your thinking style doesn't mean simply "thinking happy" or practicing positive thinking. There are tons of books, magazines, and late-night infomercials touting the power of positive thinking ("every cloud has a silver lining"). These sayings make it seem as if the world is a rosy and wonderful place, where all of life's problems melt away against the warm glow of positive thoughts. No one can argue with success, so if positive thinking works for you, keep up the good work. However, most people find that simply repeating positive thoughts is neither believable nor enough to change their behavior. For example, saying to yourself: "Each day can be a little better, each and every way" is hard to accept after you realize you locked your keys in the car right before an important meeting. Because what people tell themselves when they are "thinking positively" is just so hard to accept, positive thinking doesn't have much lasting effect on bowel symptoms or any other health problem.

A more useful, realistic approach is to develop more constructive thinking habits that help you identify your interpretations of a situation based on facts. Most of the time, you'll find that constructive thinking nips thinking errors in the bud before they take a toll on your health. In addition, constructive thinking skills will help you bounce back quickly from setbacks that all the positive thinking in the world can't disguise. In the next chapter, Step 5 looks at a number of different types of constructive thinking methods that will help you with your IBS.

CATCHING YOUR THOUGHTS

Now that you've learned a bit about how thoughts can help you get carried away, it's time to pay attention to the kinds of thoughts you have. After all, before you can change negative thoughts, you must first recognize what they are. At first, "catching" negative thoughts may be a challenge. If you have trouble catching your thoughts, it doesn't mean you have no thoughts or that they don't influence your reactions. It just means you need to sharpen your reaction time so you catch negative thoughts as soon as they appear.

"Thought catching" is an important skill, because it will give you another tool to reduce the physical responses that can aggravate IBS symptoms. Just as you monitor your body for physical tension, you can monitor your mind for mental tension caused by negative self-talk.

There are several ways to catch these thoughts. The first is to monitor them using the Daily Stress Worksheet as you did in Step 1. You'll find a blank Daily Stress Worksheet on page 239.

So how do you track these thoughts? When you first notice early signs and symptoms of an IBS attack (such as cramps or stomach butterflies), try to listen to any thoughts playing in the back of your mind. Even situations that don't involve IBS symptoms can give you a peek into the thoughts constantly crossing your mind. One way of getting at the thoughts you're having in a given situation is to ask yourself questions, such as: "What am I saying to myself or imagining in this situation?" or "What do I think or imagine will happen here?" The goal is to uncover a specific thought. You'll know you've hit pay dirt when your thought reveals a specific prediction or expectation about a situation.

If your thought seems too general, try to get more specific by simply asking yourself: "Then what do I expect to happen?" For example, a person caught in a heavy snowfall may find herself getting anxious as she says to herself: "I worry about driving in the snow." This thought isn't specific enough because it doesn't capture the scary thought or prediction that fuels her driving anxiety. By asking herself "Then what?" she is able to think through the thought to identify a more specific prediction that is making her feel anxious: "I worry that if I have to drive through the snow, I'll lose control of the car and get into an accident." In other words, what makes the situation scary is the worry (the prediction) about getting in an accident while driving through the snow.

Focus on Your Thoughts, Not Your Feelings

When it comes to "catching" your thoughts, it's important to distinguish between your thoughts and your emotions. In other words, if you want to change your thought patterns because you're worried about something you expect will happen, don't focus on how you may feel when something happens. Focus on what prediction or expectation a situation triggered. Here's an example: Let's say that giving a speech is a situation that you usually find really difficult, and so you want to track the way you think about it. What's the first thing that comes to mind when you think about giving a speech? If you say: "I'd feel nervous!" you may be right, but that's an emotion or feeling, not a thought. *Feeling* nervous won't necessarily happen if you're able to change the way you think about giving a speech.

You really need to find out what it is about the speech that *makes* you feel nervous. Your thoughts about the situation will give you a good clue as to why you would feel nervous in a specific situation. What do you think will happen during the speech that will make you nervous?

Once you dig a bit deeper, you may realize that you're afraid of making mistakes in your speech or tripping over your words, and as a result the crowd will not understand you. The initial belief, then, is not an emotion (your anxiety), it's the prediction or expectation that you'll embarrass yourself in front of a crowd.

The good news: Just as most people can crank up the emotional machinery of high anxiety by thinking scary thoughts ("What if I fail the test . . ." "What if I say something stupid . . ."), we have the power to reduce or prevent too much anxiety by tweaking the way we think.

Start Simple

Life is full of any number of daily pressures. Take a moment to think about the hassles you face. Don't worry if they seem like little things: a baby crying during a movie, an unexpected bill, a bad haircut, an invitation to a party where you don't know anyone. No situation is too minor for discovering how passing thoughts trigger our reactions.

What specific thoughts crossed your mind when you lost your keys, got a late start to work, woke up late, burned the toast, or found out the babysitter was canceling at the last minute? Catch those thoughts so you can jot them down later. Even routine daily activities provide good material for tracking your thoughts on the Daily Stress Worksheet. For example, when you sort through your daily mail, have you ever found yourself jumping to the conclusion that an important-looking letter contains bad news before you open it? This is the type of "little worry" that can teach you a lot about how you react to situations.

Another way of detecting automatic thoughts is to use your reactions as a clue. Many people with IBS find that when they feel physical pain or they're upset, they make very specific predictions or interpretations about the situation. These thoughts make up an internal dialogue that is expressed in the "What if . . ." or "If only . . ." statements discussed earlier. For example, Sue's chest pains trigger an almost immediate automatic thought: "What if I'm having a heart attack?" If Sue were to work backward from the physical chest pain to her concerns about having a heart attack, she could catch the scary thought that seemed to flash by so quickly.

Once you've snagged a negative thought, you can size it up and examine whether the thought fits the facts. Worries aren't always based on facts! If the available facts don't support your thoughts, you can tone down your reactions by considering alternative ways of thinking. For example, many people with IBS worry that they'll have an "accident" when they have a sudden urge to go to the bathroom in a public place. This would be anxiety provoking for anybody—but how do you know for sure that you'll lose control of your bowels? While it's true that accidents do happen, the overwhelming number of times that people feel a sudden urge doesn't result in an accident. If you think about how many times you've made it safely to the bathroom and how many times you've had an accident, it's probably not even a close contest. When you look at the evidence, having an accident isn't the sure thing that it seems at first glance.

Think about the number of times you've had a sudden urge to go to the bathroom in the past. Now think about how many times you've worried that you'd lose control of your bowels before reaching the bathroom. How many times have you made it safely to the bathroom without incident? When you consider how many times you've had an urge but never had an accident, you'll see that the odds of having an accident are very low—certainly much lower than your initial estimate. By looking at the evidence, you can tone down your negative self-talk and the tension it creates before it triggers a gut reaction.

In the next chapter, you'll learn constructive thinking skills to help you respond realistically to an event, before the thought triggers a reaction. This learning process is not very different from learning any other thinking skill. As a third grader, learning to multiply 2 x 3 took some thought and maybe even a bit of finger counting. As an adult, multiplying numbers comes automatically—just as the habit of constructive thinking soon will be.

TO-DO LIST

- Continue using the Daily Stress Worksheet to monitor IBS-related situations and reactions. Pay special attention to your moment-to-moment thoughts before, during, and after IBS attacks or any other challenging situation. Write down these thoughts in detail under the third column.

- Do mini practice of the quick relaxation countdown exercise (pages 92-93) throughout the day. As soon as you start to feel more tense, use those stressful feelings as a cue to concentrate on slow, smooth, deep breathing. Track your progress using the Relaxation Training Worksheet.

LEARNING TO THINK MORE CONSTRUCTIVELY

Danielle was driving down the highway one day when she suddenly felt her stomach tighten. "What's this pain?" she asked herself, starting to panic. "Is it something serious? An ulcer? Stomach cancer? I wouldn't be having these symptoms unless there was something wrong!" All morning her mind raced with worries about possible stomach problems her doctor hadn't diagnosed. In fact, her worries didn't stop until after she'd had a bowel movement. As she was walking out of the bathroom, it dawned on her that she was now beginning to think more clearly. Maybe getting herself so worked up was fueling her symptoms!

Danielle is just beginning to realize that her thoughts play a vital role in her IBS symptoms. She's starting to see how as soon as she starts having a few symptoms, her mind takes off in a million different directions at once, getting more frantic as time goes on. Soon her thoughts feel out of control and her symptoms get worse with each passing minute—a direct link between worrying about symptoms to the point of making them worse.

In Step 4, you learned how to become more aware of the role that your thoughts play in digestive health. In high-pressure situations, your first thought is often the most extreme, *not* the most accurate or useful. The sooner you learn how to identify negative thoughts, the sooner you can replace them with the more useful ways of thinking that you'll learn in this chapter.

Learning to think more constructively takes patience and practice, just like any other skill—whether it's riding a bike, driving a car, or learning to ice skate. But in some ways, modifying the way you *think* is an easier thing to do than learning any of these other skills. That's because people tend to make two very specific thinking errors that trick us into believing events are more threatening and overwhelming than they really are:

• Jumping to conclusions
• Blowing things out of proportion (catastrophizing)

With this step of the program, you'll learn how to get a handle on your tendency to jump to conclusions—just like Danielle was doing. Then in the next chapter (Step 6), you'll learn how to handle the habit of blowing things out of proportion (catastrophizing).

JUMPING TO CONCLUSIONS

You jump to conclusions when you overestimate the chances that something bad or unpleasant will happen, even if the actual likelihood is either uncertain or relatively low. Another term for this is "thinking the worst," and it's a pretty common thinking style. It's exactly what happened to Danielle, who tends to leap to the wrong conclusion—such as assuming a stomach pain is cancer. Of course, not every IBS flare-up can be easily traced to what you ate, thought, or felt. Some attacks seem to come out of the blue without any obvious trigger. In these situations, the goal is to keep a lid on your reactions so they don't aggravate symptoms and spiral out of control.

Obviously, if you think something bad is going to happen, you're going to feel more anxious—and since jumping to conclusions can increase your tension, it also can aggravate gut reactions. As you saw in Danielle's case, even in challenging situations your first thought in reaction to a bowel symptom (or other problem) is only one of many possibilities. In most situations, there are many ways to look at the same problem. You don't have to treat life as a game show where the goal is to be the first one to come up with the answer! The goal is to have the *right* answer, and this requires thinking about all of the possible explanations in a situation.

Because extreme thoughts can lead to extreme reactions, looking for alternative ways of seeing things can turn down the volume on your responses. Looking for alternatives doesn't mean looking at life through rose-colored glasses and countering negative thoughts with positive affirmations. (Most of the time, positive thinking just isn't very believable.)

Looking for alternatives means considering whether there are other possible ways of seeing the same thing.

You're guilty of jumping to conclusions if you find yourself saying things like:

- If I say no, she'll be mad at me.
- My stomach problems won't ever get any better.
- If I ask my boss for time off, she'll say no.
- I'm the worst in the class.
- When my husband's late coming home from work, I just know he's been in an accident.
- I'm going to blow this.
- Everyone at the party will look better than I do.
- I won't know what to do.
- I've offended my friend because she hasn't returned my phone call.
- I won't be able to do it.

Examine the Evidence Step by Step

We tend to jump to conclusions when the outcome of a situation is either uncertain or less certain than we'd like. For example, Jim has to give a 10-minute overview of the new sales-team projections to the home office, but he hates to speak in public. When he worries that his presentation won't go well, he's basically estimating that the chance of a poor performance is 100 percent.

It's certainly *possible* that he'll perform poorly. But is failure the *only* possible outcome? Isn't it also possible that he'll do a fine job—or at least good enough to get the job done? By assuming he *will* fail, he isn't considering other outcomes that are at least as likely to occur.

You can modify unhelpful thoughts through a simple four-step process:

1. Identify your unhelpful thoughts.

2. Calculate the initial odds.

3. Examine the evidence about your unhelpful thought.

4. Update the odds.

Identify your thoughts To overcome unhelpful ways of thinking, you must first identify your specific unhelpful thoughts during a difficult situation. You may find that identifying your thoughts is a bit like swatting a fly—they both move too fast to capture. If this is the case, try looking for even subtle changes in what you're feeling to provide helpful clues to what you're thinking—feelings such as a knotted stomach, tight shoulders, or clenched jaw. Or you may notice emotional feelings, such as anxiety.

Use these feelings or sensations to ask yourself: "What am I thinking right now?" or "What am I expecting will happen?" If you're anxious, there's a good chance that you're expecting the worst. Asking yourself these questions can help reveal the unhelpful thoughts connecting the situation to your physical reactions.

The type of situation also may provide clues to identifying your thoughts. Just as there are "traps" on the highway designed to catch speeders, some high-pressured situations are "thinking traps" where your brain moves so fast that you make thinking errors. Uncertain, new, or unpredictable situations are good examples of thinking traps where your brain is quick to go beyond the facts and jump to conclusions.

When you jump to conclusions, you arrive at the most catastrophic conclusion. Do you find that you worry as a way of dealing with situations over which you have little control? We all like to be in control of situations. The unknown can make us feel vulnerable and powerless. Sometimes we react to the uncertainty of life by worrying because it's the only option available to us. It's almost as if we think that if there's nothing we can actually *do* about a situation that has already happened or one that we envision happening, we can at least worry about it. In this case, worrying is your brain's way of mentally treading water—it might not help you get anywhere, but at least you feel like you're doing something! The problem is that worrying as a response to uncertainty isn't particularly helpful and causes more problems than it solves.

You may find that worries are more likely to appear in specific situations, such as with:

- Family members (partner takes a business trip, kids go off for an overnight)
- Performance/evaluation (taking a test, making a speech, being interviewed)
- Work (facing deadlines, taking on new responsibilities)
- Day-to-day chores (having company over, cleaning, traffic)
- Financial pressures (current or future expenses)
- Health problems (yours or family members)

What specific situations can trip you up? Take out a piece of paper and jot down some of your ideas. You may want to compare this list to the situations you wrote down on your Daily Stress Worksheet. If you can identify high-risk situations where you're likely to fall into a "thinking trap," you can plan ahead and take steps to avoid getting caught up in the vicious circle of IBS.

If you find it hard at first to identify what was going through your mind before having a reaction, start off with the statement: "I worry that . . . " and answer something like "I worry that . . . I botched the report." You can see that the "I worry that . . . " technique reveals a specific, concrete automatic thought, which is expressed as a prediction or expectation.

Calculate the initial odds Having identified automatic thoughts that may be working against you, the next step is to calculate the odds that the negative event that you predict will happen. In most cases, people initially assume that there is a 100 percent chance that whatever they're worried about will occur.

For example, imagine that your boss wants to see you. If you say to yourself: "Oh, no, my boss is upset with the way I wrote that Russell report," you're making a very specific and definite prediction about the reason your boss wants to see you. Rarely are things as definite as they first appear. You don't really know *what* your boss wants to discuss. There are likely other possible explanations for why your boss wants to see you, but you jump to the worst-case scenario. You treat your hunch as an irrefutable fact—a 100 percent probability.

While jumping to conclusions does reduce uncertainty, it does so at the expense of increasing your anxiety level. Remember: Extreme beliefs cause extreme reactions, so the more certain you estimate the likelihood that an event will happen, the more tension you'll probably feel. Learning that your thoughts are guesses — not reality — is one of the most important skills you can learn if you're going to get control over your symptoms.

Examine the evidence   If worry amounts to an absolute prediction that something will or won't happen, then you should be able to gather evidence supporting that worry. If a prediction can't be supported, it can hardly be considered a fact. For example, let's take Sue, who is getting ready for her mother's 75th birthday party when she feels her stomach act up. These sensations trigger automatic thoughts of "Here we go again . . . this is going to ruin everything. Now I'll never finish before the guests come." This is a good example of how the thoughts that automatically cross our mind are often predictions of future events "dressed up" as facts. Although Sue doesn't know for sure how the party will unfold, she assumes that her stomach problems mean that it will be ruined. Sue treats her guess (the party will be ruined) as a scientific fact, no less certain than that the sun will set at the end of the day.

You can challenge automatic thoughts by dissecting each one. What's the evidence supporting the worry? What's the evidence that counters it? It's often easier to focus on information that confirms your worries, so be sure to look for pro and con evidence. The trick is to get in the habit of considering whether there is any information that may challenge your worry thoughts and predictions. When we worry, we focus on one negative possibility while ignoring other possibilities that are at least as likely to occur. This makes it hard to overcome the habit of negative thinking.

The goal is to achieve a complete view by looking at *all* the evidence available to you. To do this, it is important to ask yourself some basic questions.

- What's the evidence supporting this belief?
- What's the evidence against this belief?
- Is it reasonable to assume that the negative outcome will definitely occur, given the evidence you have right now?
- Are there different ways of thinking about the event?

It's important to examine all of the facts BEFORE coming to a decision about how likely a negative event will occur. Step back and try to analyze the situation as an unemotional, uninvolved observer.

Update the odds   Now that you've gathered the evidence to support your first thoughts, you need to examine the real odds that a negative event will happen given the evidence you collected—in other words, you need to think objectively. This step can help you develop more constructive ways of thinking. Thinking more objectively can help stop your tendency to think the worst. Because extreme beliefs cause extreme reactions, changing what you're thinking about can help you feel less negative, which turns down the fire fueling gut reactions.

NOW IT'S YOUR TURN

On the next page you'll see an example of a completed Daily Thought Worksheet (you can find a blank worksheet on page 241). On this worksheet, you can identify your thoughts and look at them more constructively. The sheet has five columns.

1. In the first column, you'll briefly describe the situation in which you experience a bowel symptom or other negative reactions (frustration, tension, stress). These triggers can be internal (physical symptoms) or external (life events).

2. In the second column, write down your specific worry or thought triggered by the situation identified in column 1. This can be tough at first, because your thoughts are so automatic. Remember, a worry is a statement of what you predict or expect will happen in a specific situation. To help uncover the prediction, ask yourself: "What is it about this event that worries or bothers me?" or "In situation X, I worry that Y will happen . . ."

3. In the third column, write the initial odds that the negative event that worries you will happen. Estimates range from 0 percent (no chance) to 100 percent (definitely will occur), with a value of 50 percent reserved for events whose likelihood is uncertain. Because worries are predictions or expectations about future events, their estimated likelihood is typically high (in the 100 percent range).

4. In the fourth column, write down how you know that the event you're worried about will happen. What's the evidence for and against the thought? Remember: If you treat your thought as a fact in column 3, you have to come up with evidence. If there's no evidence, it's not really a fact and you're free to choose a different way of thinking.

5. In the fifth column, you want to update the realistic odds—the likelihood of the negative event occurring. It's okay to say I DON'T KNOW!

Daily Thought Worksheet

	0	10	20	30	40	50	60	70	80	90	100
	NO CHANCE				**DON'T KNOW**				**DEFINITE CHANCE**		

What was the event or situation? (1)	Specific worry or negative thoughts? (2)	Initial odds? (3)	What is the evidence? How do I know for sure? Consider alternatives? (4)	Realistic odds? (5)
Thinking of taking a leave of absence from job at pharmacy.	Uncertainty! I worry this is not the right thing for me to do	100%	• I really don't know what is going to happen. • Maybe I'm looking for the perfect solution, not the best one. • I could continue to work and go to school part-time (20 hours/wk). • Bottom line: I have NO evidence that this is not the right thing.	0-50%
My brother complains of bad headaches.	I worry that he has a brain tumor (like our mom had).	100%	I really don't know what his problem is. All we can do is wait for the doctor.	0-10%

STAY IN THE PRESENT

After a week of monitoring, many people are struck by how much of their thinking concerns events that exist only in the distant future. So much of our lives is spent thinking about the past or planning for the future that we miss what's happening in the here and now.

Think back to the last time you were driving down the highway—where was your attention focused? If you're like most of us, you devoted just enough attention to the road so that you didn't get into an accident. A good chunk of attention was likely focused on either where you were coming from, or where you were going—in other words, the past or future—but not much on the present. We live our lives on automatic pilot, not really being aware of what we presently are thinking, feeling, or doing. This makes it hard to live life to the fullest and take charge of situations rather than reacting automatically to them.

When your mind wanders, your body is more likely to get out of sync. Remember, that's precisely when IBS symptoms occur. Staying in the present helps keep your brain and gut working in tandem and your symptoms at bay.

One way to keep your mind from drifting is to focus your attention on what is happening *right now*. Giving your full attention to what you're doing at a particular moment without any thoughts about the past or the future is a skill. Focusing attention on the present moment means learning to experience life fully as it unfolds without analyzing, evaluating, or judging what it all means. Focus your attention on the here and now, where it belongs. As you learn to stay in the present, focus on the difference between what's happening right now and what exists only in your thoughts about the past and the future. No one knows how the future will unfold. The unknown makes us all feel uneasy. But no amount of worrying about tomorrow makes the future more certain or easier to tolerate. Therefore you can afford to free your mind of the urge to jump from one thing to another. Staying in the present and letting go means focusing on controlling the controllables, letting go of any distractions caused by worrisome thoughts, and attending to where you are right now.

SEE A PROBLEM THROUGH SOMEONE ELSE'S EYES

One way of looking for alternatives is to adopt the perspective of someone else in your situation. This tool is called role reversal, or shifting perspectives. Consider Sue, whose stomach acted up right as she was preparing for guests to arrive for her mother's 75th birthday party. Her unwanted body sensations triggered automatic thoughts of "Here we go again . . . this is going to ruin everything. Now I'll never finish getting things ready before the guests come."

Rather than jumping to conclusions and automatically telling herself she wouldn't be able to get things done, she could have asked herself: "What would I suggest to my best friend if she'd said that?" Most likely, Sue would have calmed her friend by saying something like: "You're not helping matters by getting yourself worked up. You've got plenty of time to get things ready, and you can always ask someone else for help if you get behind. Things will work out fine enough. They always do."

Looking for alternatives is a particularly useful exercise for people with IBS, because they tend to criticize themselves much more harshly than others do. At the root of such unfair self-talk is a tendency to lock in to one way of looking at things. Strong emotions affect our thinking this way.

Shifting your perspective will help you come up with alternative ways of approaching a situation so you think more clearly. Because extreme thoughts cause extreme reactions, looking for alternatives helps defuse the intensity of reactions caused by negative self-talk.

You're probably better at looking for alternatives than you may think. Let's say your friend calls and tells you she's afraid she failed an important test. It's clear she's looking for some advice. You probably wouldn't tell her that yes, she really is stupid and she probably did really poorly. Instead, you'd probably encourage your friend to look for other ways of thinking about her performance: You might say that feeling nervous after an exam is pretty normal, that she probably did better than she gives herself credit for, and besides, there's nothing she can do about the exam right now, so she should let things go. This is pretty good advice. If it's good enough to comfort your friend, it will be good enough advice for you to follow as well.

The ability to shift perspectives is an important thinking skill because the way you process information about your world is strongly influenced by your mood. When you're happy, your judgments are more positive. You see other people as more friendly and likeable, and relationships as more satisfying. When you're in a bad mood, you tend to focus on the most negative parts of life. When you feel under pressure, sad, or tense, you're more likely to view the world in the most threatening light. After all, in the absence of light, even the brightest colors look dark. Shifting positions illuminates your thoughts so you can see things more clearly.

By stepping back and looking at things more objectively, you can consider your responses from a calmer perspective. Here are some questions that you can use to help you shift perspectives:

- What if a friend were in my situation and asked me for advice? What advice would I give him/her?
- What would I say to a friend thinking the thoughts I'm having?

TO-DO LIST

- Practice recording your thoughts, focusing on thinking the worst or jumping to conclusions. Your ability to control negative thoughts will improve if you identify them right after they trigger a physical or emotional reaction.
- Use the Daily Thought Worksheet to work through the five steps of constructive thinking for five situations over the next week.
- Continue to fill out the IBS Diary.

STEP 6

BOUNCING BACK FROM ADVERSITY

Ben is an energetic 23-year-old who just graduated at the top of his class from law school. He was on track to achieve his goal of becoming a lawyer and was pleased to get an interview at one of the most prestigious law firms in Denver. The interview went better than anticipated: he was well prepared; he fielded their questions well, and seemed to get along well with even the gruffest of partners. Unfortunately, things went from good to bad at the end of the interview when, as Ben stood up to shake hands, his briefcase knocked over a coffee cup, spilling coffee all over his application file. When he tried to reach for the cup, he passed gas loudly. He wanted to hide under the desk. "This is terrible!" he thought. "There goes the job. I'll never live this down. They must think I'm such a fool."

Situations don't get much more embarrassing than the one Ben faced. What makes this so stressful is that it involves a situation over which Ben has no control. Nothing Ben can do can change what happened after he knocked over the coffee cup. In this chapter, you'll learn how to bounce back from the adversity of uncontrollable situations. Learning to tackle adversity requires understanding that many times when things go bad our first response is to blow things out of proportion or *catastrophize*. When you catastrophize, you are likely to focus on how bad an event was that actually happened. During stressful situations, people tend to dwell on how bad the situation is—on its cost or consequence. In Ben's case, he catastrophized by focusing on what other people thought of him and how those thoughts would impact his job interview. But when you blow things out of proportion, you typically think that the consequences of a negative event are more disastrous, unmanageable, and intolerable than they actually turn out to be. When you blow things out of proportion, you lose sight of your ability to prevail in the face of life's toughest challenges. Instead, your mind focuses on how bad the event was. The thinking error of blowing things out of proportion—just like jumping to conclusions—makes you feel more anxious.

How many times have you said:

- I'm never going to get over this.
- That ruins *everything*.
- I can't put up with this.
- I can't deal with that.
- I can never face X, Y, or Z.
- This is terrible.
- I can't stand this anymore.

When you blow something out of proportion, the "sound track" that plays inside your mind ("This is terrible!") is out of sync with your true coping abilities. This is because you often measure your ability to cope with negative events by how bad the event is. When you do this, you sell yourself short and underestimate your ability to manage your life. You need to recognize that how you *feel* about a situation has little to do with how well you can *cope* with it. Many people with IBS question their ability to cope with upsetting problems. However, these doubts often aren't based on fact, but on the amount of distress bad events cause.

The problem is that feelings triggered by negative events aren't a very good indicator of how well you cope. Can you think of a time when you coped with a problem even though it was upsetting? It might have been the death of a loved one, financial setbacks, the breakup of a relationship, an early life trauma, a job loss, or the sudden illness of a friend. No doubt these events were really upsetting. But when you look back at how you actually behaved in these kinds of tough situations, you probably realize that you can cope well with many stressful life events. In other words, your ability to cope with a situation doesn't go hand-in-hand with the distress it triggers. This is because your ability to cope with what life throws at you is based on the skills you have, not the emotions you feel. Knowing that you can cope with setbacks, and using the thinking skills taught in Step 6 to bounce back are as vital to your life as the oxygen you breathe.

Learning that you can cope with adversity is a key skill for keeping a lid on catastrophizing. For example, imagine you're in the middle of a nasty blizzard. Your front steps and porch are buried in snow. You may feel frustrated, but you don't collapse in a heap and say to yourself: "This snowstorm is so terrible, I'll never be able to cope with the snow!" You might grab a shovel and clear a path from the front door, listen to the radio for updated emergency information, or let the faucets drip a little to prevent the pipes from freezing. In spite of how bad the situation is, you cope with it the best way you can. Your ability to tolerate the storm isn't defined by how bad the storm is, and the severity of the storm and the feelings it brings on don't shake your ability to cope.

KEEP THINGS IN PERSPECTIVE

The best way to counter the tendency to blow things out of proportion is to keep things in perspective. This means realizing that even the worst consequences of negative events are more manageable than you may think they are at first. When it comes right down to it, even life's worst events rarely do us in—you can tolerate almost anything to some degree.

Getting a handle on your worries will be a lot easier if you base your estimates on evidence of what's *likely* to happen—not what *possibly* might happen. We make distinctions between possible and likely events all the time. For example, it's certainly *possible* that you could slip on a bar of soap and hit your head in the shower tomorrow morning. It's certainly *possible* that a car will bump into you on the way to the store. Are these events possible? Yes. Are they likely to happen? No.

The notion that events are possible doesn't stop you from taking a shower or driving to the store. Every day, your actions are controlled by knowing the difference between possible and likely events. Understanding this is crucial if you're going to take control of your worries. And luckily, worry control doesn't mean building all new skills—just sharpening those you already have.

Losing control of your bowels, getting a flat tire before work, being stuck in a traffic jam, misplacing your wallet, missing a flight—these events can cause understandable stress, but in the end you get through them and ultimately land on your feet. This is because we can cope with an amazing amount of adversity. When you think about it, your ability to endure past setbacks shouldn't make you feel more vulnerable to falling apart under pressure, but more confident that you'll survive whatever hardship tomorrow brings.

Of course, surviving doesn't mean that stressful situations won't upset you. We're humans, not robots! Anxiety, worry, physical pain, and bowel flare-ups aren't fun, but they are all part of life. Surviving means knowing that you'll weather adversity just as you've done countless times before, and will do countless times in the future. It means knowing you're resilient. You can experience discomfort and pain, and still cope with them.

A critical part of learning how to stop blowing things out of proportion is to look at the big picture and realize that managing IBS depends on your ability to talk yourself through the challenging situations without dwelling on the consequences of a negative event.

RIDE THE WAVE OF LIFE'S CHALLENGES

In part, your ability to manage bad things stems from a recognition that bad events won't last forever. However much distress you experience during adversity, the challenge is to ride out the discomfort long enough to prove that you can manage it. In effect, "decatastrophizing" is a bit like surfing. Like a wave, the intensity of adversity will crest and eventually subside. As the wave rolls in, the challenge is to maintain your balance and ride in to shore.

The time from the beginning of the event to when it peaks will vary, but ultimately even the worst events end. As a surfer on that wave, if you can hang on long enough you'll have successfully ridden it out. For example, many people who struggle with pain focus on how bad it feels, or worry that it will only get worse or intolerable. By blowing things out of proportion, they struggle against waves of adversity and are swept away by them. In fact, the worst-case scenario is rarely as horrible as you feared in the heat of the moment. A useful strategy is to "ride the wave" by reminding yourself that the problem will go away after it crests. What always happens is that eventually the event dissipates by itself. Some people who learn to ride the wave like to remind themselves: "I'm only minutes away from success!" when they're trying to manage a difficult event. Stress surfing can help you experience the rise and fall of stressful situations without being thrown off balance.

HOW TO STOP BLOWING THINGS OUT OF PROPORTION

You can learn how to bounce back from adversity by following these steps:

1. Identify situations where you're more likely to blow things out of proportion (problems or other setbacks you've already experienced).

2. Identify the specific thoughts that crossed your mind when adversity struck, and write down what you're saying to yourself.

3. Use the following questions to generate new, more adaptive, and reasonable thoughts whenever you catch yourself blowing things out of proportion:

   • What would *really* happen if X (such as an attack of pain) occurred?

   • Realistically, how bad would it really be if X occurred? Have I gotten through a flare-up before? Am I focusing on how bad things would be and not on my ability to tolerate adversity?

   • Am I overestimating how long X would last, and how uncomfortable it would be? Can I cope with a few minutes of X during my

Decatastrophizing Worksheet

What was the situation or event?	Thoughts during the event?	Questions to ask yourself •Is situation time limited? •Is it manageable? •Can I let go? Do I have a choice? •How useful is the thought? •Is it worth developing stomach problems over?	Physical sensations after asking yourself questions?	Feelings after asking yourself questions?	What did you do?
At the end of a job interview that I felt good about, I stood up to shake hands with 2 people interviewing me. As I reached over the desk, I knocked over a coffee cup and, to make matters worse, passed gas LOUDLY.	I cannot believe this! I want to hide under the desk with the dropped coffee cup. This is terrible! There goes the job! I'll never live this down. They must think I'm such a fool.	It hurt but there's nothing I can do about it now. Ride it out. Not helpful to focus on how embarrassing it is. I'm focusing on 5 seconds of a 1-hour interview which I felt went pretty well. Get the facts, which are not available now. Remind myself that I'll get through this. This is clearly not what I wanted to happen but it is not intolerable. Just hang in there. Tried to remind myself there is no saber-toothed tiger here.	Still felt very embarrassed and anxious but not panicky. Thinking objectively about it kept a lid on things, and other than a tightening stomach I surprised myself by not getting "bowels in an uproar." No diarrhea, no bloating.	Definitely anxious (who wouldn't be in same situation?), felt a bit down, embarrassed but not panicky.	Tried to regroup by thanking them again before I left. Wrote letters to the people who interviewed me thanking them for their time and emphasizing my strengths. Called my best friend who told me that she once read that the average person has gas 15 times a day! People must not have gas just when they're off work, right? I thought that was funny.

day? Have I been able to cope or tolerate discomfort in the past?

- Is it really terrible, or just not what I wanted to happen?

- Am I basing my judgment of how intolerable or unmanageable X would be on how strong my emotional response to a situation is? Can I think of a time when I coped well enough with a situation that triggered strong emotions? In other words, are my reactions a true marker of how well I cope with adversity?

- Do I know people close to me who have done okay when X happened? Am I really any less effective at coping than they are? Is it possible that the difference is in how they responded to adversity?

- If X were to happen to someone close to me, what advice would I give?

- Even if I can't control what happens *to* me, what can I do to control what happens *inside* me?

TRACK YOUR PROGRESS

Now, fill out the Decatastrophizing Worksheet found on page 242 (see sample on page 137). It is nearly identical to the Daily Stress Worksheet in Step 1. The only difference is that there's one extra column labeled: "Questions to Ask Yourself." Use this worksheet to record more useful ways of seeing things after asking yourself the questions on the worksheet.

TO-DO LIST

- Practice decatastrophizing skills over the next week by using the Decatastrophizing Worksheet.
- Continue to practice controlled breathing throughout the day by taking brief mini practices when you first notice yourself getting tense.
- Continue to track your bowel symptoms using the IBS Diary.

STEP 7

PUTTING YOUR THINKING SKILLS TOGETHER

Jim, 42, was stuffing the last piece of luggage into the van before taking his wife and two kids for a much-anticipated vacation to the beach when he glanced over his shoulder to see the darkening clouds of an impending thunderstorm. Within 30 minutes, water was pouring down in buckets, rushing down the streets, and slowing highway traffic to a standstill. "This is terrible," he muttered to himself. "The way things look now, the rain isn't going to stop till Sunday. The whole vacation will be ruined. No one will have fun. We've been looking forward to this trip for months, and this stupid rain will make it a nightmare."

So far you have learned two primary thinking skills. The first skill, introduced in Step 5, focused on curbing your tendency to jump to conclusions by looking at the facts before judging how likely something is, or looking for alternatives ways of thinking about an event. These strategies will guard against the tendency to automatically predict that something bad will happen. In this situation, helpful thinking skills include looking at all the facts before jumping to the worst-case scenario, examining the evidence, or looking for alternative ways of thinking about an outcome you predict will happen. As you control your beliefs, you'll see that your reactions become less extreme too.

The second thinking skill you learned (Step 6) is how to cope more effectively with adversity. Key thinking skills include: understanding that even the worst events are typically time limited and more manageable than we give ourselves credit for at first; learning to let go of situations over which we have limited control; and how to refrain from zooming in on the costs and consequences of life's negative events. Short of having a time machine, you can't do anything to reverse these events, but you can face them and keep a lid on your reactions by focusing on what you can do to cope, not dwelling on how terrible or catastrophic problems.

A good rule of thumb: If you find yourself predicting a future problem, either look for alternatives, or come up with evidence to support the realistic likelihood that an expected bad thing will really happen. If no evidence supports your worry, then you can afford to think in a more constructive manner. Remember, just because you don't know what's going to happen doesn't give you the green light to worry about possible misfortunes that may not necessarily occur or are out of your control. These two thinking skills were introduced one step at a time so that you could focus on learning these two techniques.

But while this approach helps build "mental muscle," it's not too realistic, because as Jim's situation shows, you don't jump to conclusions one week and catastrophize the next—you probably make both thinking errors throughout the week, sometimes at the same time. In high-pressure situations, you may find yourself engaging in both thinking errors at nearly the same time! Therefore, it's important to develop the flexibility to use both thinking skills when the situation demands it. Putting those skills together is the goal of this chapter. So there is good reason to learn how to combine the thinking skills you learned in earlier chapters so that you can work around thinking errors that occur in multiple situations.

TRACK YOUR THOUGHTS

One way to do that is to start logging your thoughts. On pages 144-145, you'll find a sample Thought-Tracking Worksheet (there's a blank form on page 243). For each situation, you should record your stressful thoughts in the first column, stating each thought as specifically as possible. Next, you'll need to classify the type of error you're making: Are you jumping to conclusions or blowing things out of proportion? You are jumping to conclusions if you find yourself predicting an outcome that hasn't yet occurred. If that's what you're doing, put a check in the second column. You're blowing things out of proportion if you find yourself dwelling on the consequences of a negative event that already happened. If so, check the box in the third column.

In the fourth column, you'll need to come up with a more constructive challenge to your thought by asking yourself a series of questions. These questions can help you generate a more constructive challenge to your thought, which you can then jot down in the last column. In the last column, mark whether the negative event that you expected came true or not.

Questions to ask yourself if you're thinking the worst:

- What's the evidence supporting this thought?
- What's the evidence against this thought?
- How do I know for sure that the event will definitely occur?
- Is there a different way of thinking about the event?
- What would I tell my friend if he or she was thinking the same thing?

Questions to ask yourself if you're blowing things out of proportion:

- What would really happen if X occurred?
- How bad would it be if X occurred?
- Am I focusing so much on how bad an event is that I'm not thinking about my ability to get through it? Have I been able to cope with discomfort in the past?
- Is it *really* terrible, or just not what I wanted to happen?
- Do I know other people who have done okay even when X happens? Am I really any less effective at coping than they are?
- If X happened to someone close to me, what advice would I give?
- Even if I can't control what happens to me, what can I do to control what happens inside me?
- How useful is this thought right now? Will this thought get me what I want? If not, can I just let go? Do I have a choice?

TO-DO LIST

- Use the Thought-Tracking Worksheet to record negative thoughts. Identify them as either examples of jumping to conclusions or blowing things out of proportion, and examine their validity using the questions on page 142.

- Continue to practice controlled breathing through the day by taking brief mini practices when you first notice yourself getting tense.

- Continue to track your bowel symptoms using the IBS Diary.

Thought-Tracking Worksheet

Trigger Situation	Initial Worry/Thought	Type of Thinking Error	
		Jumping to Conclusions	Blowing Out of Proportion
At 3:30, boss told me she needed me to make changes to final report before we could present it to board of directors this evening.	Is she crazy? — why did she wait till the last minute to let me know? I will never get this report done in time for the board meeting Why do I stay in this job? I worry I won't get it done like she wants before deadline	X	

Questions to Ask Yourself

·Evidence
(how do you know for sure)?
·Alternative viewpoint?
·Usefulness of belief?
·Can I shift perspective?

When I say I'll never get it done, I am jumping to conclusions.

I've been in same situation before and came through before. Part of me thrives on the pressure.

I can't afford to think the worst. For the next 1.5 hours, my attention needs to focus on getting the report done.

I'll have plenty of time to think about ways to prevent this mess from happening again — but not now!

NO

Whew!–got the report done by 4:40 p.m. Making changes to the report was easier than I first thought.

STEP
8

SOLVING PROBLEMS
EFFICIENTLY

Sue and Ellen are sisters who live in Chapel Hill, North Carolina, love horses, and both have sensitive stomachs that give them occasional IBS symptoms. But in other respects they are as different as night and day. Sue is a headstrong, impulsive woman who describes herself as a "bit of a control freak." Not one to like surprises, she leaves nothing to chance. She will lay in bed the night before a steeplechase competition thinking about every possible thing that could go wrong. "Expect the worst, hope for the best" is her motto. The longer she thinks about the competition, the tighter her stomach is tied into a knot of discomfort. Ellen, by nature calm and even-tempered, doesn't feel weighed down by worries about future events. She chooses to keep her mind from wandering too far into the future and lets go of things she can't do anything about. Ellen's IBS triggers aren't worries about the future but a tall cola and good rack of ribs at her favorite BBQ restaurant.

By now, you've probably noticed that bowel problems don't always occur at random—instead, they're often triggered by unpleasant events or circumstances. Some triggers can be physical, such as eating one too many spicy chicken wings, hormonal changes, or an infection. Other triggers—such as Sue's—can be psychological; they occur when you are faced with a problem you *can't* control. Many times, it's these daily hassles that overwhelm your coping abilities, irritate your gut, and aggravate IBS symptoms.

Of course, not everyone who experiences the same type of problem will necessarily develop bowel symptoms. ***This is because it's not the problem itself, but how people handle the problem, that often determines their reactions.*** The ability to make good decisions during a stressful situation is an important skill, because it can increase your sense of control and improve the quality of your life. On the other hand, if you're not very good at solving problems, you'll find this can worsen stress, undermine performance, and cause needless frustration.

For people who suffer with IBS, problems of daily living can aggravate bowel symptoms. Although these day-to-day problems may seem minor, it isn't always easy or possible to solve them. In this chapter, you'll learn step-by-step techniques to help you manage these problems of daily living.

HOW DO YOU HANDLE PROBLEMS?

People handle problems in many different ways. Which of the following sounds like your style?

- Are you more likely to approach problems as challenges to be solved, or do you approach problems more apprehensively, seeing them as personal threats that you'd rather avoid at all costs?
- Do you detect problems early on and give yourself time to put together a game plan with the best chance of success? Or do you sweep problems under the rug until they become overwhelming?
- Do you tackle problems head-on by applying the most promising solutions, or wait for a perfect solution that never comes?
- Do you try to fix every problem, or are you ready to admit that for some problems, there's nothing you can do?
- Faced with a problem, do you first think about the costs of not solving it before separating the issues, examining the facts, and reaching a decision?

LEARNING PROBLEM SOLVING ONE STEP AT A TIME

Solving life's problems involves strategy. Good problem solving involves a series of specific thinking and decision-making steps carries you from defining a problem to reaching a solution, with the most efficiency and the least amount of stress.

1. Define the problem. The first step in solving any problem is to define exactly what the problem is. When defining a problem, be as specific as possible, because it's much easier to solve problems that are concrete and well defined than those that are broad or vague. Overwhelming problems should be broken down into smaller, more manageable issues. This is critical to efficient problem solving. It may be helpful to ask yourself the following questions:

- What's the problem?
- What is it about the situation that bothers me?
- What do I want to happen?

Think about a problem you faced recently. Now, describe the problem in clear, specific, concrete language. It doesn't have to be elaborate.

2. Determine how fixable the problem is. Once you define the problem, you may be tempted to solve it — but like it or not, we can't always solve all the problems we face. Good problem solving often comes down to knowing the best approach for dealing with problems that can and can't be solved. Taking action to solve a problem is a good response when the problem is fixable. Many problems that stress us out don't lend themselves to an immediate solution. They are either uncontrollable or less controllable than we'd like.

Research shows that people with IBS tend to have a distinctive way of approaching difficulties geared toward "fixing" problems, no matter how controllable they are. Do you try to solve problems without first thinking about how fixable they really are? Think about difficulties you've had solving problems. In retrospect, was the problem you tried to tackle fixable and under your control?

A "can-do" spirit is a real plus if it helps keep you going until a solution is reached. However, it can be stressful to try to fix an uncontrollable problem. Therefore, efficient problem solving requires you to ask yourself some basic questions:

- Is this problem fixable right now?
- Do I have control or influence over this problem right now?
- Am I the right person to tackle this problem?

• Is it going to be possible to do this?

We often assume that the correct answer is yes to each of these questions. Take a moment to review a problem you have in light of these questions. You'll probably find that some of the most stressful situations can't be changed. The way you answer the questions above sets the stage for the remaining problem-solving steps, so make sure you answer the questions honestly. If you don't, it can cause you a lot of unnecessary aggravation. Don't let a preference for being in control influence your answers.

Let's say you're caught up in a traffic jam a mile from a meeting scheduled to start five minutes ago. It really doesn't matter that you would like to be on time. As you watch the car in front creeping along, you recognize the difficult truth: You have no control over being late. Once you determine whether the problem is fixable, you can tackle it by adopting the strategy that gives you the best chance of coping. Worrying about being late isn't going to get you to the meeting any faster.

3. Match the problem to the best coping response. There are two types of strategies people use to handle stressful situations: *problem-focused* and *emotion-focused* methods. With problem-focused strategies, you take concrete steps to change the situation itself. It's an action-oriented coping strategy geared toward eliminating or fixing the source of a problem. For example, if you were worried about an important exam, using a problem-focused strategy might include:

• Forming a study group with other students to review the exam material
• Scheduling a meeting with the teacher to clarify areas of confusion
• Asking friends who took the course for advice on what to expect

What happens if you can't do anything to eliminate or fix a problem? Some sources of stress are invariably uncontrollable and just can't be fixed. Trying to solve an unfixable problem will leave you frustrated, stressed out, and miserable.

Handling problems that can't be fixed calls for the second type of coping strategy. That's where an emotion-focused coping strategy comes in. Just because problems can't be solved doesn't mean you have to suffer from them. Dealing with unfixable problems just calls for a different method of coping called emotion-focused strategies. Let's say after you took the exam, you found yourself worrying that you didn't do well. There's nothing you can do about the test until the teacher hands out grades next week. At this point, no amount of worry will make your actual grade any better. Your only option is to adopt a coping response that limits the emotional impact. You might go to a movie, hang out with friends, go for a run, or read a book. These are examples of emotion-focused coping methods. They don't fix the problem, but they help soften its emotional impact. Examples of emotion-focused coping methods include:

- Looking at the situation in a new way (reframing)
- Reinterpreting the meaning of the situation
- Getting support from family or friends
- Taking a deep breath and calming down
- Accepting the situation, resigning yourself to an unchangeable outcome ("I can't dwell on things I can't change.")
- Letting go
- Adopting a "so what" approach

There's no single coping solution that works best in every situation. The best coping response depends on first asking whether you can or can't do anything to fix a problem, and then matching your answer to the best coping method. Problem-focused coping work best in situations where something can be done. Emotion-focused coping work best in situations that have to be accepted. Negative emotional reactions to uncontrollable events are best handled by changing the way you think about a situation. This approach can help control your reactions without changing a situation that may be beyond your control.

Stress occurs when the amount of control you really have over a problem doesn't match the method you've chosen for coping with it. This finding lends scientific support to the basic message of the well-known Serenity Prayer: "Give me the serenity to accept the things I cannot change, the courage to change the things I can, and the wisdom to know the difference."

4. Brainstorm. Once you clarify the type of coping method the problem calls for, the next step is to brainstorm a list of potential solutions. The more solutions you can develop, the more likely you'll arrive at one that will work the best. Try to think of as many options without considering how plausible they are. Don't worry about considering options that may seem unusual, weird, or funny. The important thing at this step is increasing your mental flexibility so that you don't lock yourself into a single option that may not be the best one.

5. Choose an option and act on it. Once you've identified a number of possible options, select the best one. Think through the implications of each option. You can narrow down your choices by first eliminating the solutions that are obviously not workable, either because they're too risky, unrealistic, or too difficult to carry out. Then, use the following questions to evaluate the remaining alternatives in terms of their potential effectiveness, efficiency, and side effects.

- Will this option improve the situation?
- What are the pros and cons?
- How much time and effort does this option require?

After you compare the options, decide on the one that is likely to resolve the problem in the most satisfactory way. If you have come up with a number of potential solutions and carefully thought through their implications, the best option is usually pretty clear. The best option doesn't have to be a perfect solution–just "good enough." Sometimes, several options seem equally attractive, and you can combine them to form a better solution.

Once you decide on an option, act on it. You don't have to stick rigidly to the option you've selected; if it doesn't resolve the problem, you have the luxury of turning to a number of other options that you identified in the brainstorming process. Remember, problem solving is an ongoing process, not a one-shot, all-or-nothing deal.

6. *Evaluate the results.* How did your approach work? What actually happened? Did you find yourself spinning your wheels pursuing an option that in hindsight had little chance of working? What was most and least helpful? What changes would be beneficial at this point? After you have given the approach a fair trial, does it seem to be working out? If not, consider what you can do to beef up the plan, or give it up and try one of the other options. It may be necessary to repeat the step before a complex problem is solved.

PROBLEM-SOLVING TECHNIQUES

To solve problems efficiently using the strategy just discussed, try to make use of the following techniques: start simple, plan and rehearse, be reasonable, focus on changing yourself, not others, make a contract with yourself, expect some failures and learn from them, reward yourself, keep at it.

Start Simple

Now that you've learned how to solve problems, begin with a small problem; you can work up to larger problems later. If you want to test your belief that saying no to a friend will jeopardize your friendship, begin by seeing what happens when you refuse a simple request. A series of small victories will build your confidence so you can tackle larger problems later.

It's important to look for opportunities to improve your problem-solving skills, regardless of whether they are related to bowel problems. Any problem without an obvious solution gives you a chance to strengthen your problem-solving skills.

Plan and Rehearse

Figure out in advance what you might say and do to address the problem. Run your game plan by a friend. Then, before you take action, clearly imagine yourself carrying out the task. Try to picture yourself as clearly as possible in your mind's eye. Hear your voice and watch yourself as you visualize yourself take action. The more clearly you can picture yourself carrying out the task, the better (reread Step 3 if you need to refresh your memory on visualization). If you clearly imagine yourself doing something, this mental picture is likely to help you achieve your goals by shaping your actions.

Be Reasonable

It can be difficult to test a solution. Don't expect perfection the first time. Give yourself credit for each step you take. Expect ups and downs along the way.

Focus on Changing Yourself, Not Others

It's much easier to change your behavior than someone else's. If you find that your options require changing another's behavior, it may be a clue that you have unrealistic expectations of what you can change. Taking responsibility for other people is often a prescription for frustration.

Make a Contract with Yourself

Make a firm commitment to experiment with a solution on a specific day, in a specific situation. Then stick to it!

Expect Some Failures and Learn From Them

Developing more efficient problem-solving skills takes time, practice, and patience. Don't be discouraged if your efforts fall short at times. Failure is important to the learning process. Asking yourself what went wrong when you failed can teach you how to be better prepared the next time.

However, make sure you learn from your mistakes, or you'll be wasting your time. Did you have control or influence over the problem? Were you the best person to tackle the problem? Were you drawn into solving a problem by taking on the problems of somebody else? Was this problem worth solving?

Reward Yourself

Have you ever heard that "you have to break some eggs to make an omelet"? When it comes to problem solving, failure can help improve your problem-solving skills. Rewarding yourself for having tried can get you through periods of discouragement and reinforce your commitment to problem-solving skills training. Give yourself a pat on the back for a job well done.

A more formal way to reward yourself is to use a system that links completing the problem-solving steps with something pleasurable. An effective reward is something that makes you feel good and is readily available after you finish the steps. The reward doesn't have to be expensive or extravagant. Sleeping in late on the weekend, buying yourself a cappuccino, taking a hot bath, renting a video, reading a trashy novel, or spending some time with good friends are effective rewards that fit easily into most schedules and budgets.

Keep at It

Practice is the key to changing behavior. A solution that feels awkward and difficult the first time will become easier with practice. Remember, you're learning a new set of skills, and any new skill is bound to feel awkward at first. Self-defeating activities may feel normal, but they aren't helpful. If the problem-solving exercise feels awkward, that's probably a good sign. If you don't feel a bit awkward, it could be a sign that you're relying on seat-of-the-pants problem solving.

The Problem-Solving Worksheet can help you work through all the problem-solving steps (see the sample on page 157). There's a blank form on page 244.

TO-DO LIST

- Remember that the best problem-solving response is based on how controllable a problem is. Emotion-focused responses work best for uncontrollable problems, while solving problems is best for controllable problems. Think about the problems you struggle with over the next week. Are you matching the true controllability of a problem to the right problem solving response? If so, good job. If not, notice how frustrated, stressed out, and overwhelmed you are likely to get.

- Learning more flexible problem-solving skills is tough work that requires some practice and perseverance. Behaviors that feel awkward at first will become easier and more natural the more you practice. So keep at it long enough to see the benefit.

Problem-Solving Worksheet

Key Questions to Ask Yourself	Problem
What is the problem? Be specific, clear, and concrete •What is bothering me? •Why is it a problem?	Got phone message from friend asking if I could pick up her daughter at ballet. I have a MD appointment at same time. Specific problem: Conflict between my schedule and friend's request.
How much control do I really have over this situation? •Am I taking on too much responsiblity for things I can't control? •Am I ignoring aspects of the problem that are under my control? •Is the goal under the scope of what I can do?	Initial thought: "If I don't do it, who will?" On the other hand, as much as I'd like to help, picking up her daughter is really not my responsibilitiy.
What can I do? Be specific, clear, and concrete •Write down all the possible options (even if they seem silly or impossible). •No criticism or judging •Think quality not quality •Match the option to type of problem (controllable vs. uncontrollable)	1. Don't call back and pretend I never got the message. 2. Cancel MD appoint and reschedule. 3. Tell her "how dare you treat me like a chauffeur" (I'd never say that!). 4. Tell her that I can't because I have a MD appointment at the same time.
Think it over •What could happen with each option? (Consider the type of problem, time required, costs involved, effects on me personally, effects on others.)	If I cancel MD, I have to wait another 3 mos.– already waited 3 mos. for this appt. No need to get nasty. If it were someone else in same situation, I'd suggest explaining that she was just busy at the time she wanted daughter picked up.
Make a decision •Pick a solution that's best for me (consider the consequences). •Don't wait for perfect solution–pick one that's "good enough."	I'll just have to say that while I'd like to help out. I just can't do it. After all, she was just calling to see if I was available. It's not like she called with expectation that I would pick daughter up.
Now do it •Figure out what you need to carry out a solution and do it.	Be up front. Don't let my emotions make the decision for me. What are my priorities here? My health or working out my friend's scheduling problems?
How did it go? •Am I satisfied? •If not, what else could I do?	Even though I thought I'd disappoint her, she said she understood. Anyway, ballet teacher will drop off her daughter on way home.

STEP 9

CHALLENGING CORE BELIEFS

Mara, 47, was up late last night celebrating her birthday, and got up at least a half hour late for work the next day. A long-time IBS sufferer, she found herself stuck in the bathroom three days a week, trying to have a bowel movement. Each minute that passed made her more tense, because tardiness was frowned upon at her computer programming firm. Mara immediately started thinking the worst: "I'm going to be late for my 9 o'clock meeting, If I'm late, the others won't like it. My supervisor is going to start wondering if I'm cut out for this job. I can't deal with this pressure," she went on. "Maybe I should never have accepted this job in the first place. If only I'd stayed at my old job, this wouldn't have happened."

As she finally left home and got into her car, the bloating and stomach cramping worsened while driving. It was rush hour, and every mile was sheer agony. As she checked the clock on her dashboard, she felt her head pounding hard, sweat droplets across her forehead, and her stomach muscles tightening. "Now I'll be even later," she agonized, "because I won't be able to join the meeting until I go to the bathroom."

As you can see, Mara was really running on "autopilot," with one automatic thought after another racing through her head and affecting her body. In earlier chapters, you learned to identify automatic thoughts and replace them with more constructive ways of thinking. As you will see in this chapter, these automatic thoughts are often influenced by our beliefs, which in many ways are as unhelpful and inaccurate as our thoughts.

In earlier chapters, you learned to identify automatic thoughts and replace them with more constructive ways of thinking. Now, we'll focus on identifying the beliefs that trigger automatic thoughts. While thoughts and beliefs seem a lot alike, they have important differences as Mara discovered.

Thoughts are the moment-to-moment internal dialogue you carry on with yourself during the day. As you drive through the supermarket parking lot, this dialogue may sound something like: "Sure is busy today . . .

hope I didn't leave my grocery list at home. Oh, there's a parking space, I'll grab that one!" Waiting for your doctor, you may say to yourself: "I hope she gets here soon . . . I have to get to work by one." Getting dressed in the morning, you may look in the mirror and say to yourself: "I don't really like how this shirt looks on me. I should have worn the blue one."

Beliefs are far more general than thoughts. Beliefs cut across different situations, reflecting your overall attitude, outlook, or assumptions about life. Thoughts are snapshots of how you see things at a single point in time, whereas beliefs are the camera lens through which you see the world. Some beliefs are like a wide-angle lens that lets you see the big picture. Others are more like a close-up lens that magnifies an image in great detail. Just as the type of lens makes a difference in how a snapshot comes out, your beliefs can influence the content of your moment-to-moment thoughts.

Beliefs are shaped by years of life experiences. The belief that "You should be respectful to elders" prompts you to open the door for an older person. Other beliefs, however, can be a source of strain and tension. People with IBS typically struggle with three core beliefs:

- Perfection is possible
- I expect approval
- I have control

EXPECTING PERFECTION

No one's perfect. Yet many people with IBS expect perfection from themselves. Perfectionism isn't necessarily bad; athletes, artists, and teachers often achieve high levels of performance because of the high standards they set for themselves. This type of perfectionism involves a healthy pursuit of excellence. In "healthy" perfectionism, people can lower their standards when a situation requires it.

People with IBS often strive to meet very high standards in everything they set out to do. Because of a constant pressure to achieve, they have trouble adjusting their standards to fit the situation. Perfectionists often define their self-worth based on their most recent accomplishments. Perfectionists rarely feel that they've done their job well enough and, as a result, their accomplishments rarely provide satisfaction. They have trouble tolerating mistakes and are hard on themselves when things don't go just right. They criticize themselves excessively. Perfectionists get more upset over mistakes because they're afraid others will judge them as harshly as they judge themselves. As a result, they're reluctant to ask for help to correct problems, and they have a strong urge to cover up mistakes, even normal ones we all make.

Excessive concern over making mistakes can be a source of stress, worry, and anxiety. Perfectionism also can create other problems. It can force you to put things off, avoid activities where there's a potential for making mistakes, and invest excessive time getting things done just right. If you're critical of yourself for making mistakes that you'd ignore in others, if you hesitate to take on new challenges for fear of failure, or if you worry how well you're doing, you may be expecting perfection. The drive toward perfectionism is fueled by specific beliefs. Do any of these beliefs sound familiar?

- People will probably think less of me if I make a mistake.
- If I'm worthwhile, I must be the best at all times.
- If I don't do well all the time, people won't respect me.
- What I accomplish is never quite good enough. I can always do better.
- I must give more than 100 percent in everything I do or else I'll be mediocre or even a failure.

EXPECTING APPROVAL

Not everyone will approve of what you do. In fact, there's probably someone who would disapprove of just about anything you do. But many people still believe that they must be accepted and approved by everyone, even though it's impossible. If you find yourself worrying about what others are thinking about you, or if you often hesitate to say no because of what someone else might think, expecting approval may be generating stress for you. A need for approval is associated with specific thoughts:

- I can't stand to be put down by people who are important to me.
- What other people think of me is very important.
- I can't find happiness without being loved by someone else.
- Everyone must like me.
- My family will be upset with me or disapprove of something that I do.

THE ILLUSION OF CONTROL

The last common core belief involves the illusion of control. This belief tricks your mind into thinking in a specific, unrealistic way. People with an illusion of control feel responsible for everybody and everything that comes their way. Their sensitivity to the needs of others piles the weight of the world on their shoulders. Everyone at work counts on them. Their friends depend on them. They assume responsibility for others' happiness. Their self-talk often includes the refrain: "If I don't do it, who will?" Because there is no shortage of other people's problems, they often feel exhausted by the end of the day and have little left in the tank to fuel their own needs. And because they take on more than they can handle, they feel guilty when they don't come through for others.

The illusion of control hinges on an overinflated belief in your ability to fill others' needs and the expectation that you're responsible for filling those needs. The illusion of control fuels the flame of worry because worry often occurs when you feel the need to control the future.

People who have an illusion of control have a hard time tolerating uncertainty. As much as you'd like the world to unfold in a predictable manner, life is full of surprises — some good, some bad. People who can't tolerate uncertainty have trouble accepting the fact that it's part of everyday life. Does this sound at all like you? If you answer yes to any of the following, you may have difficulty tolerating uncertainty:

- Does uncertainty make you feel more uneasy or tense?
- Do you feel frustrated if you don't have all the information you want to make a decision?
- Do you believe that you should always look ahead so as to avoid surprises?
- Do you believe you should be able to organize everything in advance?
- Do you describe yourself as a bit of a "control freak"?

An intolerance of uncertainty leads to more "what if" thinking in many situations. If you're intolerant of uncertainty, you tend to focus on all the bad things that might happen. Even if most of these bad things have almost no chance of occurring, you'd still dwell on them. Therefore, all possible outcomes and their consequences will be imagined. This sets into motion a series of reactions that includes worrying and increased physical reactions.

CRACKING THE ICEBERG

These beliefs—perfectionism, expecting approval, and the illusion of control—aren't always easy to spot. It may not have dawned on you that any of your thoughts have anything to do with these beliefs, but they do. It's as if your thoughts and beliefs are like an iceberg, with just a tip above the waterline. Your thoughts are the more readily identifiable tip of the iceberg, and your beliefs are lurking beneath the surface. If you want to destroy an iceberg, you can't just chip away at the tip. You have to get at the stuff below the surface—the core beliefs—before you can destroy the iceberg.

Getting Beneath the Surface

You can identify your core beliefs by taking one upsetting thought or worry and asking yourself a couple of simple questions: "If this thought is true, why is it upsetting me?" The core belief may not become so apparent the first time you ask yourself this question. If it isn't, that's a sign that the belief is far below the surface. With each negative thought you identify, you should repeat the question: "If this thought is true, what would be so upsetting about that?" until you generate a chain of negative thoughts. As you dig deeper, you should repeatedly ask yourself this question until you uncover a thought that illustrates one of the core beliefs described earlier.

Let's explore finding a core belief. Say you're at home on a Saturday afternoon, and a group of your friends stops over unexpectedly. Almost right away, you start to feel anxious and your gut tightens. Your automatic thought begins with this thought to yourself:

I can't believe this. My place is a mess and I'm in no shape for company.
(Suppose my place *is* a mess, what would it mean or say about me?)
↓
That would mean they'll think I'm a slob.
(Suppose I am a slob, what would it mean or say about me?)
↓
That would mean they'll think less of me.
(Suppose they do think less of me, what would it mean or say about me?)
↓
That would mean I'm not the person I should be.
(Suppose I'm not the person they thought I was, what would it mean or say about me?)
↓
That would mean that I'm not perfect.

This example shows how repeatedly asking yourself: "Suppose X, what would it mean or say about me?" triggers a cascade of thoughts that flushes out a core belief that involves perfectionism. The more negative thoughts you generate, the closer you get to uncovering what the core belief is.

When practicing this exercise, make sure each of your answers captures a belief or assumption, not a feeling or emotion. In the example, notice how each question brings out a specific thought—"they'll think I'm a slob" or "they'll think less of me"—not an emotion the person was feeling. If you focused on the emotion, you wouldn't be able to pinpoint the core belief supporting automatic thoughts.

Pinpointing core beliefs is a bit like peeling an onion layer by layer until you reach the center. As each layer of thought is peeled away, a more extreme thought is uncovered. Just as peeling onions may bring tears to your eyes, uncovering successive negative thoughts can trigger more extreme reactions. You can see that the sequence of statements leading to the core belief is stated as fact when they are really guesses ("they will think less of me"). Sometimes the search for the core belief is obvious after asking yourself one time: "If this thought were true, what would it mean or say about me?" Sometimes, the questioning process takes longer to pinpoint the core belief. After you have listed a series of negative thoughts, ask yourself what the core belief is.

LOOKING FOR ALTERNATIVES

Once you've identified your core beliefs, you can challenge them by considering different ways of thinking about the same event or by testing the accuracy of your predictions. Here are three practical strategies that can help you view situations in more useful ways:

- Reversing positions
- Reframing thoughts
- Identifying the usefulness of the belief

Reversing Positions

This strategy refers to seeing things from someone else's point of view. Ask yourself: "What if a friend were in my situation and asked me for advice?"

Think about your friend's situation objectively. What advice would you offer? What choices might your friend have? Try to see the situation as your friend would. How might this person approach the problem? When things get overwhelming, remember a new spin of the Golden Rule: *Say not to yourself what others wouldn't say unto you.*

Reframing Thoughts

Reframing means changing the way you think about an issue. Just as you might reframe a picture that clashes with your furniture, you can reframe your thoughts. By reframing, you ask yourself: What other ways of viewing this situation are there?" This question allows you to see situations from a more manageable, useful, or tolerable perspective. A situation always can be seen in several ways, any of which could be true. A glass can be either half full or half empty.

When you're under stress, your perspective narrows and you tend to see only one view. Reframing a situation allows you to consider different ways of looking at the situation. S-T-R-E-T-C-H your mind by coming up with other explanations besides the first one that popped into your head. Very often an alternative way of seeing things can tone down your reactions to situations caused by extreme thoughts.

How Useful Is the Belief?

When you focus on the consequences of a situation, you forget that some belief —regardless of how accurate or important they are—are just not very useful. For example, no one would argue with a trauma surgeon who says: "If I make a mistake, my patient could die and the family would be devastated." Is such self-talk accurate? Yes. Is such self-talk useful? No. You want the surgeon to focus her attention on the surgical procedure, not the worst-case scenario should the surgery go badly. In other words, "What if . . ." thoughts aren't very useful. Looking at the usefulness of a thought is a particularly helpful tool for dealing with perfectionism and intolerance of uncertainty.

One strategy for challenging the need for certainty is to ask yourself questions about how useful the belief really is. If you were cleaning your basement and came across a box filled with old Cat Stevens records, legwarmers, love beads, and leisure suit—what would you do? Would you throw them away after realizing they've outlived their usefulness? You can just as easily discard negative thoughts by asking yourself whether they're worth keeping. Here are some easy challenges for examining the usefulness of negative thoughts:

- How useful is it for me to believe X?
- Have I learned to tolerate other uncertain events in the past? If so, can I learn to tolerate this one?
- If I can't increase my certainty of what's going to happen in the future, can I at least better tolerate the unknown by examining the usefulness of my beliefs?

TESTING THE ACCURACY OF PREDICTIONS

After you've used these three techniques to challenge a stressful belief, you may want to challenge this belief further by testing the accuracy of your predictions. This skill is also called reality testing.

First, predict what you think will happen in a situation. Let's say you have to give a speech, and you hate public speaking because you're sure your opening joke will fall flat. State your prediction: "My opening joke won't be funny." Be as specific as possible. Then test your prediction against what actually happened. Ask yourself whether the prediction came true. "Was my opening joke a dud?" "Actually, it wasn't! Everyone laughed just the right amount!"

One reason that your stressful thoughts and beliefs don't fade away is that you never give yourself the chance to look back and see whether your guesses come true. When you do a little reality testing, you find that most of the evidence you collect doesn't support stressful thoughts. By doing this over and over, you give yourself another tool to overcome the habit of negative thinking.

Here's an example of reality testing. Imagine that today you found an error in a final report but you're reluctant to mention it to your boss because you worry that she'd consider you a complainer. As you think about talking to your boss, your stomach feels a little queasy. Here's how to test the belief that bringing up a problem would be viewed as complaining: Go ahead and show your boss the problem with the report. Afterward, think about what happened. Was the outcome as bad as you predicted? Did you come off as a complainer? Was your boss put off by your comment? Did she appreciate hearing about the problem? Did your stressful thought come true? People don't often test beliefs because doing so involves experiencing some tension long enough to test the accuracy of the stressful thought.

Imagine gathering in front of the TV for the Bills-Dolphins game. You expect a sure win for the Bills. Even though you predict a Bills victory at kickoff, you wait till the end to catch the final score, right? You wouldn't assume that your pre-game prediction of a Bills victory is necessarily accurate when you're talking to friends about the game on Monday morning. You test the prediction against the final score. We will use this same thinking skill with everyday events.

Testing beliefs about unpleasant events can help show you that your predictions about an event are a lot scarier than the event itself. While testing your predictions may be a little unsettling at first, it's a powerful way of demonstrating that stressful thoughts and beliefs are typically inaccurate guesses. Reality testing also shows you the value of looking at objective evidence and putting things into perspective. As you gather objective evidence to counter your stressful thoughts, you'll ultimately feel less stress and more confidence when faced with the same type of situation in the future.

Start Simple

Test the accuracy of your predictions with a simple exercise. If you want to test your belief that saying "no" to a friend will jeopardize your friendship, begin by saying no to something that's easy to refuse.

- *Plan and rehearse.* Figure out in advance what you'll say and do. Rehearse beforehand. It can be helpful to have a friend review your plan with you.
- *Be reasonable.* It can be awkward to try something new. Change is difficult; don't expect your test to work perfectly the first time. Give yourself credit for each step you take.
- *Make a contract with yourself.* Make a commitment to conduct your test on a specific day, in a specific situation. Stick to it.
- *Evaluate the results.* Study what happened. What did you think would happen? What actually happened? What are the results of your test? Did you prove your stress-generating belief wrong?
- *Keep at it.* Practice is the key to changing stress-generating beliefs. Exercises that feel awkward and difficult the first time will become easier with practice.

NOW IT'S YOUR TURN

Now you can try getting beneath the surface on your own. The easiest way to identify core beliefs is to examine your worksheets for common themes. Do any patterns emerge from your monitoring? Do some thoughts keep coming up over and over? Is there a common theme to these thoughts, such as: "I should do everything perfectly" or "If there's a problem, I should be able to fix it."

You can use the Challenging Core Beliefs Worksheet to examine underlying beliefs related to stress that aggravate bowel symptoms or other problems. (See sample opposite; a blank worksheet is included on page 245.)

The format of the Challenging Core Beliefs worksheet is similar to the Thought-Tracking Worksheet you completed earlier. The main difference with this worksheet is that after identifying your automatic thought, you'll uncover its underlying core belief. The following tips can help you think through the automatic thought to the point where you reveal the core belief.

1. Follow the thread of negative thoughts by asking yourself:

   • If X were true, what would it mean to me, or say about me?

   • If X were true, why would that be so bad?

2. As you ask these questions, move from specific thoughts to broader beliefs or attitudes about how you see yourself as a person, how you see others, or the world in general.

3. Make sure you focus on thoughts. Don't use the questions to describe your emotions or bodily reactions. For example, it may be tempting to respond to the question "What does it mean to me if I get stuck in a traffic jam?" with the statement: "I'd be angry." However, this captures an emotion (anger)—not a thought. A more useful "thought" response would be: "If I got stuck in a traffic jam, it would mean that I couldn't do what I planned on doing." By focusing on a thought instead of an emotion, you move closer to uncovering the core belief that keeps automatic thoughts alive.

4. Search for the core meaning of statements, guided by at least one of the three core beliefs of perfectionism, expecting approval, and illusion of control. For example, what core belief underlies the thought: "It would mean I couldn't do what I planned on doing"? The correct answer is either perfectionism or illusion of control. People who think they have more control over their situation than they really do or

Challenging Core Beliefs Worksheet

Situation	Thoughts	What would it say about me if thoughts were true?	Type of Core Belief •Perfectionism •Illusion of control •Expecting approval	Alternative Thought •Reversing positions •Reframing •Usefulness of thought
Loads of errands to do–checked my voice mail and a friend called needing a favor from me!	I worry about not having time to get everything done. I want to be able to do everything asked of me.	I will have to say no. I'll let people down. Friends will think they can't count on me. They will look down on me.	Expecting approval	I can't be everything to everybody ALL of the time! Not helpful for me to predict what my friend may think. If the situation were reversed, my friend would understand.

who have perfectionistic beliefs may have a hard time when their goals are blocked.

5. Choose a more useful replacement thought to challenge the negative thought. For the example above, which of the questions/statements below could help you work through the thought: "It would mean I couldn't do what I wanted to do."

- Is there an alternative way of looking at the situation?

- Is this really the worst thing in the world?

- Can I see this problem as part of life? After all, everyone falls short of their goals sometimes.

- How would I encourage someone else to think about the same situation?

- Am I overstating how much control I have in this situation?

- How useful is thinking this way?

- Regardless of what I want to happen, is there anything I can really do about it? If I can't do anything about it, can I just accept or resign myself to it? Do I have any other choice?

- Even if the worst happens, can I remember that it will pass and be over soon? Can I just accept that's the way it is?

TO-DO LIST

- Use the Problem-Solving Worksheet to work through any problems.
- Fill in the Challenging Core Beliefs Worksheet to challenge underlying beliefs related to stress that aggravates bowel symptoms.
- Continue to fill out the IBS Diary.

STEP 10

IDENTIFYING SKILLS THAT WORK FOR YOU

When Sandy's youngest brother Jim got laid off, he asked her for some cash to fix his car. Even though Jim and Sandy were always close, she knew he was irresponsible and tended to rely on her to bail him out of jams. As she heard him ask for the money, she felt her stomach tighten with that familiar pang of apprehension and pain. "All I could think about was that if I don't give him the money, who will?" Her other brothers never pitched in when needed, leaving Sandy in a position to bail Jim out. "I worry he won't pay it back and I'll be out the $100 he thinks it'll take to fix the car. And if he doesn't pay the money back, I won't have money to pay for soccer camp this Friday. Why should I disappoint my son to bail Jim out one more time? My son has been looking forward to this camp all winter. Why am I always the one that my family turns to for money?"

Usually, Sandy would have allowed her stress to spiral out of control, triggering bouts of diarrhea and anxiety. In fact, that was her very first impulse until she realized the value of using her physical symptoms as a cue to apply the skills she had learned to manage her symptoms. "Wait! She thought. "It doesn't have to be this way!

It was time for Sandy to take stock of what she had learned and what she needs to do to maintain the changes she had worked hard to achieve. And time for you, too! The first steps of this program focused on using relaxation strategies to control physical changes that produce body tension. You began this program by learning how to breathe and how to create a deep state of relaxation. Like any skill, this takes time and practice, practice, practice.

Then you learned several strategies to control the mental tension that can aggravate IBS. One set of skills was designed to help you stop jumping to conclusions and blowing things out of proportion during high-pressure situations; you learned strategies to analyze the accuracy of self-defeating thoughts and substitute more constructive ways of thinking. The second set of skills was designed to improve your ability to tackle real problems, which, if unresolved, can be a source of stress.

As you've practiced the skills, you've probably found some strategies more helpful than others. Some people may find that looking for alternatives and using logic are particularly helpful, while others prefer problem solving and reversing positions. Identifying the strategies that are most effective to help you fine-tune those techniques and include them in your daily routine. Spend a few minutes reviewing the strategies in the box on page 176, and think about those you prefer.

IF YOUR SYMPTOMS HAVEN'T IMPROVED

If you haven't noticed a significant improvement in your bowel symptoms, don't be discouraged. It takes time to seize control of symptoms. You've had these symptoms for months, if not years. If you're just learning the steps, it may take another month or two before you start to see an effect. But if you continue using these skills, chances are you'll be rewarded.

Continue using the worksheets you've found helpful to identify factors that might contribute to your bowel symptoms. You also may want to review worksheets from the past to see if there has been a change in the pattern of your bowel symptoms over time.

You can continue to improve your skill in managing your symptoms. If you're thinking this means more work, remember that it took much more effort to learn these skills in the first place. As you continue to hone your symptom-management skills, you'll find they become almost automatic.

Some who have used this program have found it helpful to periodically review their strategies. Investing a little extra time every few months can prevent a flare-up from turning into problems in the future. It might help to schedule the following activities every three months:

• *Relaxation practice.* Spend two days practicing your relaxation skills. This will help you see if you're still able to produce a deep state of relaxation.

Identifying Skills That Work for You

Review the skills below and indicate how useful you found each strategy. Feel free to skip the ones that you didn't have a chance to try, or to add strategies you discovered on your own.

Managing Physical Tension

	Not Useful		Moderately Useful		Very Useful
• Tracking physical symptoms	1	2	3	4	5
• Abdominal breathing	1	2	3	4	5
• Mini relaxation	1	2	3	4	5
• Your own strategy	1	2	3	4	5

Managing Mental Tension

	Not Useful		Moderately Useful		Very Useful
• Tracking thoughts	1	2	3	4	5
• Challenging worries	1	2	3	4	5
• Decatastrophizing	1	2	3	4	5
• Looking for alternative views	1	2	3	4	5
• Testing predictions	1	2	3	4	5
• Problem solving	1	2	3	4	5
• Uncovering core beliefs	1	2	3	4	5
• Your own strategy	1	2	3	4	5

• *Track symptoms.* For a few weeks, keep tabs on your symptoms using the Daily Stress Worksheet. Try to get a handle on any symptom patterns. This information will help alert you to your reaction to situations, and what corrective action to take.

• *Reread the first chapter.* It focuses on how bowel problems can spiral out of control; this will also help you anticipate and take action to control future symptoms. You've had these symptoms longer than 10 weeks, so reading through the material once or twice may not be enough. These details may need to be reread before they become an automatic way of thinking and behaving.

IF YOU HAVE A SETBACK

At some point, you may find that your symptoms reappear because of changes in your life. For example, stress at work or home may increase, your schedule at work or home may change dramatically, or some other factor influencing your bowel symptoms may change. Don't despair! It will be easier to regain control of your bowl symptoms than it was to control them the first time around.

Detect Cues Early

It's most important to tackle problems early. Because bowel symptoms are often part of a chain of events triggered by situations, thoughts, body sensations, and emotions, it's important to detect the cues as early as possible. Don't wait until things build up so that taking control seems an uphill battle.

Treating bowel symptoms is a bit like pulling weeds in your garden. The sooner you take steps to get at their roots, the sooner they're gone! To help you detect cues early, think about what specific situations or conditions are most likely to bother you. Many people with IBS have specific high-risk situations where they are more likely to have a flare-up: shopping, at the movie theater, driving a car, attending a social gathering, dealing with deadlines or new responsibilities at work, handling conflict, or health worries. Other people with IBS may find that strong emotions such as anxiety or frustration are their Achilles heel. Once you know what specific situations can trip you up, you can watch for them, and get ready to use your coping strategies.

Work the Program

Given how common digestive problems are in the general population, symptoms are bound to reappear every once in a while. Remember, two out of every three people without IBS experience bowel symptoms in stressful situations. So if your stomach acts up every once in a while, it doesn't mean there's something wrong. How you react to symptoms will make the difference in whether bowel symptoms are simply a flare-up or become a chronic problem.

Times of high stress and upheaval may be red flags for when your bowel symptoms are particularly likely to erupt. Treat high-stress situations just like you would when you see a red flag on the highway: S-L-O-W D-O-W-N. Step back and ask yourself: What's going on here? What is it about this situation that is making me react this way right now? Use this information as a guide for what strategies to focus on.

Feeling a buildup in body tension? Time to get back to doing relaxation exercises. Feeling keyed up or worried about something specific? Probably a good clue to work on thinking constructively. Feeling overwhelmed and tapped out? There's a good chance that problem-solving strategies can help you restore a bit of balance in your life.

Keep in mind that you already have the skills to manage IBS more effectively. If you get a bit rusty, you just need to review the materials and sharpen your skills. You won't have to learn them all over again.

Keep a Healthy Attitude

How you respond to flare-ups influences their long-term course. If you become discouraged and give up or think you failed, regaining control of your bowel symptoms may be difficult. However, if you approach flare-ups as an opportunity to learn, examine what might have changed, and experiment with skills to regain control, any setbacks will be only temporary.

ON TO THE REST OF YOUR LIFE!

While reading this book, you've learned many skills for managing IBS. You've learned how to relax in order to control the physical tension that causes bowel symptoms. Then you learned how to control the mental tension that aggravates bowel symptoms.

Now that you've completed the 10 steps of our IBS treatment plan, we hope your confidence in your ability to manage your bowel symptoms is growing. Keep this book to review as needed. Remember, with the skills available to you, you can control your IBS instead of letting it control you. On pages 247-249 is a list of resources that may be helpful to you, including: patient advocacy groups; government, educational, and professional organizations; and newsletters and books.

Good luck!

PART THREE

ADDITIONAL
SELF-CARE SKILLS:
DIET AND MEDICATION

FOR MANY PEOPLE, LEARNING TO CONTROL IBS SYMPTOMS can be achieved by mastering the skills in the 10-step treatment plan. Others find that the value of these skills can be strengthened by making other lifestyle changes in their diet and medication. Part Three provides an overview of the role of diet and medication in managing IBS. Whether you have just been diagnosed with IBS or have a complex case for which behavioral skills are not enough, you will find this information useful in navigating the other treatment options available to you. Part Three leads off with a clear, concise review of the role of diet in the treatment of IBS. The most accurate and up-to-date information about diet issues is balanced with practical tips that you can put to use immediately to maximize your control over symptom flare-ups. The medication chapter provides important information about the most common medications used to treat IBS—from laxatives to antispasmodics to the new serotonin modifier drugs designed specifically for IBS. This chapter offers unbiased, science-based information about how the different categories of medications work, their benefits and side effects, and their track record of success with IBS symptoms. A useful chart synthesizes all this material in a handy, all-in-one reference.

THE ROLE OF DIET IN CONTROLLING IBS

Tom is a 30-year-old lead guitarist for a popular local rock band, whose IBS symptoms began "further back than I can remember." While he was always able to work around constipation, it had become more of a problem over the past four months. His bowel movements gradually decreased to three a week and when he did have one he typically strained to complete it. No matter how many times he had a bowel movement, he felt there was something there that he hadn't evacuated. In addition to constipation, bloating, straining, and stomach cramps were taking a toll on his work. On more than one occasion, he was late arriving to the club because he was in the bathroom. His bandmates were getting so annoyed that he consulted a gastroenterologist. After undergoing a number of diagnostic tests to rule out anything serious, Tom was diagnosed with IBS. As a first step, his doctor outlined a number of simple diet changes Tom could make to feel better. While these changes didn't cure his IBS problems, he gradually noticed less straining and an increase in the consistency and frequency of bowel movements for the first time in years.

This book seeks to give you a road map for learning how to take active control of your IBS symptoms. The previous 10 chapters focused on teaching you 10 behavioral tools for combating the self-defeating thoughts and behaviors that can aggravate flare-up symptoms. As you work through this book, you will likely find yourself moving closer to your goal of managing your IBS symptoms more effectively.

As with most maps, this one offers alternative routes to the desired destination. Some people like Tom may find that their preferred route toward symptom self-management involves making lifestyle changes that focus on their dietary patterns. In the United States, dietary changes are the most frequent recommendations physicians first make to their IBS patients, particularly when symptoms are milder. The popularity of dietary change reflects its low cost, convenience, and the strong link many patients make between the timing of their symptoms and what they eat.

Because of the link between symptoms and food intake, many IBS patients suspect they have a biological disease that renders them physically intolerant of certain foods or ingredients. There are many types of unpleasant food reactions. These include food allergy, food intolerance, and food aversions. These terms are often used interchangeably. This can be confusing because each term refers to a discrete medical condition with its own underlying cause, signs and symptoms, and treatment. The goal of this chapter to help you understand the meaning of these terms, how they relate to IBS, how specific foods and food ingredients can trigger GI symptoms, and what simple dietary changes you can make to gain added control of IBS symptoms.

FOOD ALLERGIES

Food allergies are usually caused by the protein component of an offending food. Proteins provide the building blocks for muscle, bone, skin, hair, and many other tissues. In people with food allergies, rather than being digested as most proteins are, some of the food protein is absorbed intact from the intestine. After the protein enters the bloodstream, the body's immune system mistakenly identifies it as a harmful substance (called an antigen) and unleashes an army of chemicals (such as histamine) to defend the body. The release of these chemicals can cause a wide range of symptoms including: swelling of the lips, tongue, and throat, wheezing, vomiting, nausea, headache, stomachache, abdominal cramps, and itchy hives. In extreme cases, the allergic reaction can include *anaphylactic shock*. When this happens, blood pressure drops severely; water rapidly leaves the bloodstream, causing severe swelling; and bronchial tissues swell dramatically. This causes the person to choke and collapse. Anaphylactic shock is fatal if not treated immediately. Symptoms of a food allergy can occur within a few minutes to two hours of eating or even touching a food to which one is allergic. Symptoms can range from mild to severe, and the amount of food necessary to trigger a reaction varies from person to person. If a true allergic reaction is suspected, people with allergies are advised to avoid the offending food itself and any foods or drinks that contain the food.

Food allergies are more common in children, most of whom outgrow them by the time they enter school. In children, the most common food allergies are to cow's milk, eggs, wheat, and soy. In adults, the pattern is somewhat different, and the most common food allergies are to tree nuts (almonds, walnuts, pecans, etc.), fish, shellfish, and peanuts. Experts estimate that only 1 to 2 percent of adults in the general population are truly allergic to certain ingredients in food.

Researchers have sought to determine whether food allergies are more common among IBS patients than in the general population. In one study, 30 percent of subjects suspected they had a food allergy because their symptoms began shortly after eating. Subjects then underwent standard allergy testing to determine what food substance triggered an allergic response. Only 1 to 5 percent of the subjects had a positive allergy test. These findings suggest that the frequency of a food allergy in IBS patients is similar to adults in the general population. Other researchers have found that more than 50 percent of IBS patients have a positive allergy test. However, the foods that provoke positive results during allergy testing are not the same ones they identify as causing their symptoms. This testing pattern is called a "false positive" because individuals with positive results do not turn out to have a true allergy to the problem food. If you have a suspicious allergy test, remember that it is not all that uncommon among IBS patients, it doesn't necessarily mean you have a true food allergy, and rarely explains the stomach problems of IBS patients.

FOOD INTOLERANCES

A food intolerance is a more common set of food reactions whose symptoms mimic those of a food allergy but arise for different reasons.

Whereas a food allergy is an abnormal response to a food triggered by the immune system, food intolerance is often caused by a chemical deficiency in the digestive system. With food intolerances, the body either lacks or has a shortage of enzymes that break down a portion of the offending food into absorbable components. The unabsorbed foods remain in the digestive system, causing the symptoms of bloating and cramps. There are other differences between food intolerance and allergy. Even a small amount of a food may trigger physical symptoms for someone with a food allergy, whereas food tolerances are "dose related"—that is, people with food intolerance may not have symptoms unless they eat a large portion of the food or eat the food often. For example, people with intolerance to milk may have no problem drinking a cup of coffee with milk or a single glass of milk, but become sick if they drink several glasses of milk in one sitting. But people with a milk allergy may have GI symptoms after consuming a small amount of milk or milk products that does not typically trigger symptoms in people with food intolerances.

Lactose Intolerance

The most common type of food intolerance is lactose intolerance, affecting 25 percent of Americans. As you learned in the first chapter, people who are lactose intolerant have an insufficient amount of lactase, an enzyme that lines the gut and helps digest milk sugar (lactose). The deficiency makes it hard to digest milk or milk products without experiencing stomach cramps and diarrhea. The severity of symptoms depends on many factors, including the amount of lactose a person can tolerate and a person's age, digestion rate, and ethnicity. The incidence of lactose intolerance is very high among non-Caucasians. Lactose intolerance occurs in equal proportions in IBS patients and the general population, arguing against the notion that IBS is due to lactose intolerance. That said, some IBS patients may be truly reactive to dairy products even if they are not physically intolerant to lactose intake. If you cut down on dairy products to manage IBS symptoms, make sure your diet includes enough calcium from other sources to be nutritionally balanced. Avoiding or drastically limiting consumption of dairy foods reduces intake of several key nutrients such as calcium, which is important for building and maintaining strong bones and reducing the risk of osteoporosis.

Fructose and Sorbitol Intolerance

A smaller percentage of people are physically intolerant to foods sweetened with fructose or sorbitol. Fructose is a naturally present fruit sugar used as a sweetener and found in candies, soft drinks, fruit drinks, honey, and jams. It is called a fruit sugar because it is found in some fruits such as cherries, dates, and grapes. Fructose is also found in some root vegetables (beets, onions, artichokes) and wheat. In sufficient amounts, fructose can cause diarrhea and other GI symptoms such as gas, bloating, and stomach rumbling. Even though IBS patients have more severe GI symptoms than the overall population, their rates of fructose intolerance are similar. This makes it hard to point to fructose intolerance as the cause of IBS. However some IBS patients identify foods heavy with fructose (carbonated beverages, fruit drinks, sports drinks) as dietary triggers for diarrhea.

Sorbitol is a sweetener used in many sugar-free or "dietetic" candies, cake mixes, syrups, and other foods, as well as in some medicines like cough syrups. Sorbitol has fewer calories than regular sugar because it is not completely absorbed by the body. As a result, it travels undigested to the large intestine. There, bacteria break down the food, which can cause gas, abdominal discomfort, and/or diarrhea. Up to half of adults in the general population can experience stomach problems at sorbitol doses as low as 10 grams. While sorbitol does not cause IBS, it can aggravate some IBS symptoms in some individuals.

FOOD AVERSION

So, you may be thinking if IBS is neither a food allergy nor a food intolerance caused by chemical deficiency, how do I make sense of my gut's reaction to what I eat? Some of the most common food reactions aren't "hardwired" physiological reactions but are acquired as a result of a combination of factors. These factors include your learning history, temperament, social environment, beliefs, diet, and biological makeup—such as the sensitivity of the gut or the balance of neurotransmitters like serotonin levels in brain (see the next chapter for more information about serotonin and IBS). Any combination of these factors can interact to influence our taste for and reactions to food.

One powerful influence is our learning history. If eating a particular food, such as a warm, soft, gooey chocolate brownie is followed by positive feelings and a sense of satisfaction, we are likely to develop a learned preference for chocolate brownies. The opposite is also true. If eating a brownie is followed by a bout of diarrhea, we may learn to associate brownies with stomach problems even though the relationship between ingesting them and having diarrhea may be coincidental (i.e. not due to the ingredients of the brownie). This is a learned response called food aversion. If the food aversion is strong enough you might find that even the sight, smell, or memory of a brownie is powerful enough to make you as sick to your stomach as the brownie itself. Food aversion is an important survival mechanism that works much like the protective "fight-or-flight" response you read about in the first chapter. The ability to develop a food aversion allows us to select nutritious foods while protecting us from munching on harmful substances (e.g., poisonous berries) whose toxins kick in long after ingestion. If you never learned that a food was dangerous and shouldn't be eaten, you would make the mistake of eating something that could harm you. Sometimes food aversions are "overlearned" in that they are associated with foods that aren't physically dangerous or life threatening. A food aversion that develops following ingestion of nonpoisonous foods like a rich bowl of fettuccine alfredo or a spicy bean burrito just doesn't have the same survival value as the rancid turkey hiding in the back of the fridge since last Thanksgiving.

One's learning history may also help explain why IBS patients report such wide variation in their dietary triggers. For some people, spicy or fatty foods are a surefire way to the bathroom. For others, raw vegetables like cabbage, broccoli, and Brussels sprouts do them in. Others find that they can eat these foods without any problem, but pay a price when they consume carbonated beverages, foods containing caffeine (chocolate, tea, coffee), or foods sweetened with sorbitol or fructose. So many different foods affect different individuals with IBS so differently that there is no simple, clinically proven diet for IBS. However, there are important dietary guidelines that you can easily incorporate into your lifestyle to keep a lid on some of your symptoms.

Another factor that influences food aversion is bowel sensitivity. Because people with IBS symptoms have a GI system that is supersensitive to stimuli like food, they can have colonic contractions sooner after a meal than people without IBS. This exaggerated gut reaction (called the gastro-colic reflex), particularly in individuals who are keenly aware of bodily cues associated with harm, may set the stage for acquiring a food aversion. This learning process may help explain the very real connection some patients make between the onset of their symptoms and the timing of meals, partic-ularly large ones containing rich, gassy, fatty foods. Because IBS is neither a toxic reaction to harmful food like a food allergy nor a food intolerance caused by a chemical deficiency, IBS patient's difficulty tolerating specific foods may be partly understood as a learned food aversion subject to a host of environmental, biological, and psychosocial factors.

AN ELIMINATION DIET

One way of identifying the association between a food and a patient's symptoms is using a elimination diet. This involves systematically eliminating any suspect foods from your diet for several weeks until your symptoms subside. You then begin to reintroduce the foods one at a time, in increasing doses over several days. If an unpleasant reaction occurs, the offending food is withdrawn from the diet again, and the symptoms allowed to clear before another food is tested. While time consuming and costly, this technique can help pinpoint which foods and at what dosages cause adverse reactions. Elimination diets are often used to identify food intolerances. It is believed that a person is intolerant to a food when symptoms reappear when the offending food is reintroduced to their diet. Once the problem foods have been pinpointed, your doctor can advise you how to modify your diet to avoid a recurrence of symptoms. Because elimination diets exclude from your diet foods with nutritional value, it is recommended that they be carried out under the direct supervision of your doctor to ensure that your diet provides adequate nutrition.

The general principles of an elimination diet can be useful in identifying food triggers of IBS patients. You may find that your symptoms fluctuate as you eliminate and reintroduce specific foods into your diet. This is not a flawless method. Psychological factors can affect the diet's results. For example, you may be more likely to report a stronger negative reaction to a specific food that you expect will cause you problems. Your expectations may also influence whether you have a positive response to an elimination diet. In other words, beliefs can have at least as powerful an effect on how your body responds to food as its ingredients. The results of an elimination diet may be hard to interpret in IBS patients whose symptoms often fluctuate over time. Because IBS is so complex, changes in symptoms over time are not necessarily due to dietary changes per se. In other words, it is difficult to tell whether the occurrence of IBS symptoms is caused by reintroducing a food during the elimination diet or by the natural fluctuations in the course of IBS. About half of IBS patients describe themselves as being intolerant of at least one food. Dairy products and wheat are common sources of food intolerance.

KEEPING A FOOD DIARY

Most adverse reactions to food are discovered through trial and error to determine which food or foods triggers symptoms. You may be asked to keep a food diary to record what you eat at each meal and when you get symptoms, and then put on your detective hat to look for relationships between foods and symptoms. A food diary can help you discover trends in foods and symptoms. The form on page 246 has been designed to let you record important information about your diet and symptoms.

The sample food diary on the next page shows what one day of a person's food diary might look like. Copy the form on page 246 and use it to record the foods you eat each day as well as when your IBS symptoms begin. To get the most out of a food diary you want to record some basic information.

- *Track everything you eat throughout the day.* Don't limit your entries to main meals. Record everything you eat such as condiments (dressing, cheese, mayonnaise) or the donut hole you grabbed at the office. As you learned earlier in the book, sometimes the smallest "taste" of food packs a powerful punch on your gut. Write down the type of food, how it was prepared (e.g., fried, baked, steamed), how much you ate (¼ cup or ½ cup), when you ate, any symptoms that followed, their severity, when they occurred, and medications and other treatments you took to manage them.
- *Record in real time.* Don't rely on your memory to remember what you ate while you are laying in bed at the end of the day. Research shows that our memories aren't good enough at the end of the day to

Food Diary

Name Julie Lecavalier

Day June 8

Food and Amount	Time	Symptoms	Severity of Symptoms 1 2 3 4 5 Low High	Time	Treatment or Medication
Breakfast Coffee, black–1 cup, 1 slice, wheat toast w. jam, banana-1 medium, low-fat yogurt-1 cup	7:30 am				
Mid-morning Snack Bottle of water	9:30 am				
Lunch Cheeseburger w. 1 slice bacon; 1tbsp ketchup & mayo, corn chips-3/4 bag, Coke-12 fl. oz	12:00 pm	Bloating Crampy, gassy		12:25 pm 12:45 pm	Gas-X
Mid-afternoon Snack Fat-free potato chips- 1 small bag	3:00 pm	Loose stool		3:20 pm	Nothing
Dinner Stir-fried vegs-1 cup Sesame chicken-6 oz. (wok fry) Steamed white rice-1/2 cup hot tea 2 cups	6:30 pm	Gas, bloating Urgency, loose stool		7:10 pm	Imodium
Evening Snack Small handful dried fruit/ nut mix	9:00 pm				

remember accurately everything you ate. So write it down as soon as possible after eating to ensure that the information will be as accurate as possible.

- *Be honest.* You have nothing to gain and a lot to lose by trying to look good when completing the diary. Don't worry about the cold piece of pizza you ate for breakfast. You can only get help if you record what you really eat not what you think others want you to eat.
- *Make it easy on yourself.* Carry the food diary in your pocket or purse so you can capture the information right after each meal and symptom flare-up. If you forget the diary, jot the information on a slip of paper and then transfer it to the diary later
- *Put your detective hat on.* Share your food diary with your doctor to identify foods that may trigger your symptoms. The information may unearth some patterns between your symptoms and your diet, which you can use to make different food choices in the future. For example, you can see that the person who completed the diary (opposite) linked two bouts of diarrhea to what she ate at dinner and lunch.

Any information you get is good information. If you are not successful in isolating a food culprit, don't worry. The lack of information gives you good reason to invest time and effort in mastering the behavioral skills featured in the 10-step plan. Keeping a food diary is a proactive strategy you can use to gain some control over your symptoms.

ROUGHING IT: DIETARY FIBER AND IBS

Having learned how and why specific foods can cause gut problems, you're ready to learn some simple ways to change your eating patterns to gain more control of GI symptoms. If you suffer from constipation, one dietary change you can make is to increase the amount of fiber you eat (we'll discuss diarrhea later). Diets that are low in fiber are often viewed as a common cause of constipation in the general population. For this reason, some patients can be helped with a fiber-rich diet. Unlike other food substances, fiber is the part of food that the body *cannot* digest; it is fermented by bacteria in the colon. Fiber is found in edible plant foods such as whole grains, vegetables, beans, fruits, nuts, and seeds. Animal products, such as meat, cheese, and eggs, don't contain any fiber.

One way of categorizing fiber is by its ability to dissolve in water. *Soluble fiber* partially dissolves in water and takes on a soft, gel-like texture in the intestine. Foods high in soluble fiber include oat bran, oatmeal, beans, peas, rice bran, barley, citrus fruits, strawberries, and apple pulp. Soluble fiber works like a sponge to soak up water and it is what gives oatmeal its gummy texture. In the GI tract, the absorbency of soluble fiber bulks up the size of the stool and softens its texture. This helps prevent the formation of hard, dry stool and eases their passage without straining. Insoluble fiber does not dissolve in water and passes through your digestive tract virtually intact. *Insoluble fiber* is found in whole-wheat breads, wheat cereals, wheat bran, rye, rice, barley, most other grains, cabbage, beets, carrots, Brussels sprouts, turnips, cauliflower, and apple skin. Insoluble fiber works as a natural laxative by speeding the passage of stool through the gut and out of the body. Most foods that come from plants contain a mixture of both types of fiber.

Figuring Fiber

Based on the most recent scientific evidence, the American Dietetic Association recommends that most people eat 20 to 35 grams of dietary fiber daily depending on their age and gender. The typical American eats only 11 grams of fiber each day. One reason we eat so little fiber is that our diet contains a lot of refined and processed foods (American cheese, packaged cakes and cookies, frozen dinners, or white bread for example) whose natural fiber is essentially stripped away in the food manufacturing process. The following table shows the fiber content of some common foods.

Dietary Fiber Content of Common Foods

		Serving Size	Amount of Fiber in Grams
Breads, Grains	White bread	1 slice	0.6
	Bagel, plain	4"	2.0
	Whole wheat bread	1 slice	1.9
	100% All Bran	½ cup	8.8
	Corn Flakes	1 cup	0.7
	Shredded Wheat	2 biscuits	5.5
	Oatmeal, cooked	1 cup	4.0
	Rice, brown, cooked	1 cup	3.5
	Rice, white, cooked	1 cup	0.6
	Spaghetti, Whole Wheat, cooked	½ cup	3.2
Fruit (fresh)	Apple, with skin	1 large	3.3
	Apricots	1	0.7
	Banana	1	3.1
	Blackberries	1 cup	7.6
	Blueberries	1 cup	3.5
	Dates	5	3.3
	Grapefruit, pink and red	½ cup	2.0
	Melon, cantaloupe	1 cup	1.4
	Orange	1 small	3.1
	Peach	1	1.5
	Pear	1 medium	5.1
	Raisins	1 cup	5.4
	Raspberries	1 cup	8.0
	Strawberries	1 cup	3.3
Vegetables	Beans, baked, canned, plain	1 cup	10.4
	Beans, green, cooked	1 cup	4.0
	Broccoli, raw	1 cup	2.3
	Brussels sprouts, cooked	1 cup	4.1
	Cauliflower, cooked	1 cup	3.3
	Carrots, raw	1 cup	3.1
	Cucumber, unpeeled	1 cup	0.5
	Corn, yellow, cooked	1 cup	3.9
	Lentils, cooked	1 cup	15.6
	Lettuce, romaine, raw	1 cup	1.2
	Potato, baked, with skin	1 potato	4.4
	Split peas	½ cup	8.1
	Tomato, red, ripe	1 tomato	1.5
Other foods	Meat, milk, eggs		0
	Almonds (24 nuts)	1 oz.	3.3
	Peanuts dry roasted (approx. 28)	1 oz.	2.3
	Prunes, dried	5	3.0
	Raisins	1 cup	5.4
	Walnuts, English (14 halves)	1 oz.	1.9

Source: U.S. Department of Agriculture
Note. Low sources of fiber are foods that contain less than 2.0 grams fiber per serving. Good sources of fiber are foods that contains approximately 2.5 grams of fiber per serving. Excellent sources of fiber are foods that contain at least 5 grams of fiber per serving.

Because so many foods include a healthy dose of fiber, it is not that difficult to raise your daily fiber content to meet the recommendations. If you eat two to four servings of fruit, three to five servings of vegetables, and six to eleven servings of cereal and grain foods, you should have no trouble boosting your daily fiber intake to 25 to 30 grams. All fruit and veggies aren't equally rich in fiber, though. Fruits and vegetables that are particularly rich sources of fiber include artichokes, avocados, dried fruit, baked potatoes with the skin left on, pears, and carrots.

For many people, increasing fiber intake requires making some simple changes to their eating patterns. At first, this may be easier to do at breakfast, where you have a lot of options. Simply starting the day with a serving of whole grain cereal like oatmeal or shredded wheat gives you at least 5 grams of fiber. If you top the cereal with wheat germ, raisins or other dried fruit, bananas, apples, or berries, you are well on your way to getting the recommended daily fiber by the time you head out the door. By comparison, fruit juice that is mostly sugar and water, donuts, sugared cereals, breakfast bars, or pastries alone provide virtually no fiber (less than 2 grams per serving). Many commercially available oat bran and wheat bran products (muffins, waffles) actually contain very little fiber. And they may have a high fat content that can aggravate IBS symptoms in some people. Make sure you read carefully the labels on all packaged foods (see box on page 200).

You want to spread fiber intake throughout the day at meals and snacks. Use the simple tips below to add dietary fiber to your diet:

- Choose whole grain breads and rolls over white bread that has been stripped of its fiber. Look for breads that contain 100 percent whole wheat. In North America, ingredients in foods are listed on food labels in order of their concentration in the food. Look for bread that lists whole wheat flour as the first ingredient.

- Eat vegetables raw or tender. Whether you're boiling, steaming, or microwaving, heat and humidity can break down the fiber into its carbohydrate components, which reduces fiber content. Add raw vegetables to your diet or cook them so that they offer a slight resistance when bitten into, but aren't soft or overdone.

- When possible, eat the skin of fruits and vegetables such as carrots, potatoes, apples, and peaches. By peeling the skin, you literally throw away a major source of fiber. Eating a well-cooked potato with the skin on almost doubles your fiber intake compared to eating the peeled potato; eating apple skins adds about 40 percent more fiber than a peeled apple. Leaving the skin on fruits and vegetables quickens food preparation time and increases fiber intake.

- Experiment by substituting beans, peas, and lentils for meat. Dry peas and beans and tofu (bean curd) have a lot of fiber and are rich in nutrients. Try adding a half cup of beans to pasta, soups, casseroles, and vegetable dishes. Because unprepared tofu is a rather bland tasting product, it readily takes on the flavors of the other ingredients you cook with. Try marinating tofu instead of meat in a BBQ sauce, grilling it, and serving it on a crusty whole grain baguette for a tasty, IBS-friendly dish.

- Buy fiber-rich fruits (apples, bananas, plums) and vegetables as snacks rather than cookies, crackers, or candy.

- Dried fruit also makes a great snack. It is fiber rich, easy to carry, and stores well. Because it's dried, ¼ cup is equivalent to ½ cup of fruit in other forms. Widely available dried fruits dried include apricots, apples, pineapple, bananas, cherries, figs, dates, cranberries, blueberries, prunes (dried plums), and raisins (dried grapes). Keep a package of dried fruit in your desk or bag and snack on them instead of sweets.

- Juicing fruits or vegetables removes their fiber-rich skin and membrane. Drinking juice with pulp added doesn't boost its fiber content. Make most of your fruit and veggie choices fiber-rich whole or cut-up fruit rather than juice. When possible, opt for the apple instead of the apple juice.

• Sticking to a fiber-rich diet is challenging but not impossible when you eat out because you can't readily tell what the ingredients are. Most national restaurant chains like McDonalds, Subway, Panera, Ruby Tuesdays, Starbucks, and Olive Garden offer a handful of whole grain choices like whole wheat tortilla wraps, bran muffins, fruit salads, whole wheat pasta, and whole wheat rolls. In addition to dietary fiber, make sure you factor in portion size, fat and sodium content, calories, and other nutrition considerations when making a decision about what to eat wherever you are.

Easy Does It

If you are not used to a fiber-rich diet, you may want to make these changes gradually over about three weeks because increasing fiber intake too quickly can cause gas, bloating, or discomfort. Most people experience gas and bloating when they eat gassy fiber-rich foods such as cabbage, broccoli, cauliflower, legumes (dried beans and peas), grains, cereals, nuts, seeds, or whole-grain breads. If this is a problem, you may want to try an over-the-counter digestive aid like Beano before your meal. Beano comes in liquid and tablet form and contains a sugar-digesting enzyme that helps digest the sugar in beans and many vegetables. The enzyme can break down the gas-producing sugars if taken just before eating. Beano has no effect on gas caused by fiber. Another self-care strategy is to soak the beans overnight and rinse them thoroughly. This breaks down some of the gas-causing substances, making them easier to digest.

Drink Plenty of Liquids

To reap the benefits of fiber, it is very important to drink plenty of fluids. The combination of a diet low in fiber and insufficient fluids is identified as a leading cause of constipation. Although increasing fluid intake does not necessarily help relieve constipation, many people report some relief from their constipation if they drink fluids (such as water and juice) and avoid dehydration (the loss of vital fluids and electrolytes your body needs to maintain vital functions). Liquids add fluid to the colon and bulk to stool, making bowel movements softer and easier to pass. Because fiber absorbs a lot of water, a fiber-rich diet may be constipating unless you drink plenty of fluids. If you have loose stool, it is also important to drink fluids to replace the fluids and nutrients lost through diarrhea. However, not all liquids are created equal. Caffeinated beverages, such as coffee and cola drinks, will worsen symptoms by causing dehydration. Alcohol is another beverage that causes dehydration. It is important to drink fluids that hydrate the body, especially when consuming caffeine-containing drinks or alcoholic beverages. The Institute of Medicine advises that healthy adults drink 9 cups (women) to 12 cups (men) or more of liquids each day. This may seem a bit daunting but there are some tips that can make 9 to 12 cups easy to achieve:

- Make a habit of drinking a cup of water as soon as you wake up and right before you get into bed.
- Drink water with meals and snacks.
- Instead of a coffee or tea break, take a water break.
- At parties, substitute sparkling water for alcoholic drinks, or alternate them.
- Add thin slices of orange, strawberry, lemon or cucumber to a chilled pitcher of water, so that it tastes more refreshing and makes you want to drink more of it. When you are done with the pitcher, the fruit at the bottom is a great fiber-rich snack.

In addition to water, get fluids from healthy, low-calorie beverages such as 100% fruit juice, skim or low-fat milk, or frozen juice bars (100% juice). Many foods are also good sources of fluids. Juicy fruits like oranges,

Are You Label Able?

The Food and Drug Administration (FDA) regards fiber as such an important part of a healthy diet that it requires it be listed on the Nutrition Facts of food labels along with other key nutrients and calories. Dietary fiber is listed under the total carbohydrates section of the label. It shows the amount of dietary fiber as well as the Percent Daily Values (%DVs) based on a 2,000-calorie diet. The fiber content is listed in grams and as a percentage of the daily value. The % Daily Value help you know whether the nutrients in a serving of food contribute a lot or a little to your daily intake. Food manufacturers can claim that a product is "a good source" of fiber if it provides 2.5 to 4.9 grams of fiber per serving (10 to 19 percent of the DV). The package can claim "high in," "rich in" or "excellent source of" fiber if the product provides 5 grams or more per serving (20 percent of the DV). A food that has "more or added fiber" has at least 2.5 g more per serving. If the food provides less than 5% of a % DV, it is low in fiber.

Regardless of what bowel problem you have (diarrhea, constipation, alternating), reading food labels makes good nutrition sense. If diarrhea is aggravated by artificial sweeteners, you want to know whether a sweetener has been added to a food. Look for ingredients such as sucrose, honey, glucose, molasses, dextrose, corn sweetener, fructose, high-fructose corn syrup, maltose, sorghum syrup, mannitol, fruit juice concentrate, and sorbitol. These are different sweeteners added to food. If one of these terms appears first or second in the list of ingredients, or if several of them appear, the food is likely to be high in added sugars and may be worth avoiding or used sparingly depending on your symptom profile.

grapefruit, cantaloupe, grapes, watermelon, and apples contain a large quantity of water in proportion to their weight, making them a good way of "eating" your way to your daily fluid requirement.

BEYOND FIBER AND FLUIDS

In addition to paying attention to your fiber and fluid intake, there are some other things to keep in mind as you try to manage your constipation.

Listen to Your Body

Because the timing of bowel movement can be so irregular, some constipated people suppress the urge to have a bowel movement when it is inconvenient or they are "too busy." When you have an urge, use it as a cue to find a bathroom as soon as possible. Suppressing the urge and putting a bowel movement off till later can weaken the natural signals your body relies on to move your bowels. Ignoring these cues can set in motion a vicious cycle of constipation, unproductive straining, and frustration.

Get Off the Couch

A lack of physical activity can lead to constipation, although doctors don't know precisely why. Constipation often occurs after an accident or during an illness when one is confined to bed and is pretty sedentary for a prolonged period of time. Lack of physical activity is identified as one factor that helps explain the frequency of constipation among older people. While there is limited evidence that increasing physical activity has a specific effect on constipation, general health benefits make it a lifestyle change doctors prescribe their constipated patients. Adults should strive to get at least 30 minutes of physical activity on most days, preferably daily. You don't need to become a gym rat to get the health benefits of exercise. Adding "lifestyle exercise" into everyday activities is a great start. For example, consider parking farther away in the parking lot at the mall; getting off the bus or subway one stop early and walking the rest of the way; or taking the stairs instead of the elevator.

MANAGING PROBLEMS WITH DIARRHEA

For patients with problem diarrhea, the dietary strategy for controlling IBS is more challenging than for constipated IBS patients who can add fiber to their diet to manage symptoms. Dietary fiber was once routinely prescribed for diarrhea on the grounds that it bulked up watery stool. As you will see in the next chapter, clinical studies do not show that dietary fiber is effective in reducing diarrhea associated with IBS.

In fact, too much fiber can actually aggravate IBS symptoms. For this reason, patients with diarrhea are occasionally encouraged to lower but not eliminate their intake of dietary fiber until flare-ups subside. The goal of a low-fiber diet is to reduce foods such as whole grains, most fruits, and vegetables, legumes, and seeds. Because fiber is an important part of a healthy diet, it should not be avoided altogether. Patients on a low-fiber diet are often encouraged to increase their intake of soluble (as opposed to insoluble) fiber. Because soluble fiber stays in the gut longer, it takes longer to exit the digestive system, and prevents worsening of diarrhea. Examples of soluble fiber-rich foods include carrots, apples, oranges, legumes, and oat bran. Low-fiber diets are not intended for long-term use and should be undertaken with the knowledge of your doctor. A diet low in fiber can and should be nutritionally balanced.

Generally speaking, IBS patients are encouraged to identify foods that aggravate their symptoms. This recommendation is partly based on research showing that meals stimulate contractions in the colon. Normally, this response may cause an urge to have a bowel movement within 30 to 60 minutes after consuming a meal. Because IBS patients have a supersensitive gut, the urge may come sooner and is accompanied by abdominal cramping and diarrhea. The strength of the response often corresponds to the number of calories in a meal—the larger the meal the greater the response. This suggests that *how much you eat* may be at least as important as *what you eat*. The following section will give you practical, concrete tips for reducing symptoms triggered by or aggravated by food.

The Skinny on Fat

Fatty foods are one of the most common dietary triggers of IBS. Whether it originates from vegetable or animals, fat stimulates muscle contractions in the gut after a meal. This accelerates passage of food through the intestine. Many foods contain fat, especially meats of all kinds, poultry skin, whole milk, cream, cheese, butter, vegetable oil, margarine, shortening, avocados, and whipped toppings. If you think fatty foods trigger your symptoms, there are some small, simple changes you can make that can dramatically affect the overall fat content of your dally intake.

- Eat plenty of grain products, vegetables, and fruits, which are generally lower in fat.
- Limit your intake of processed foods such as crackers, cookies, cakes, and higher fat snacks
- Limit fast food, which tends to be high in fat, salt, and calories. If you do eat fast food, check for lower fat alternatives liked grilled chicken breast sandwich without mayo; small roast beef or hamburger without cheese, garden salad with reduced fat dressing; or turkey breast sandwich. Extra meat and sauces add up to three times the calories and fat. Pass up or request smaller amounts of the high-fat toppings. Examples include bacon, mayonnaise, extra cheese, and special sauces. Instead, add lettuce, tomatoes, and mushrooms to dress up your low-fat burger.
- When cooking, broil, bake, grill, and roast instead of fry. If you sauté, use chicken broth, vegetable stock, tomato juice, or wine instead of just oil or butter.
- When eating out—select broiled, baked, grilled, or roasted menu items. Ask for reduced fat items or look for a healthy heart symbol.
- Use fats and oils sparingly. Substitute balsamic vinegar for butter on broccoli which cuts down on the fat but not the flavor. How about

apple butter on a bagel instead of a schmear of cream cheese?

- Use fat-modified foods such as lower-fat dressings and spreads.
- Choose low-fat milk products, lean meats, fish, poultry, beans, and peas to get essential nutrients without increasing fat intake.

Other Possible Food Triggers

While fatty and fried foods are common triggers, other foods can make IBS worse including: chocolate, alcohol, caffeinated beverages such as coffee, tea, and cola, milk products such as milk, cheese, pudding, and ice cream, foods containing the artificial sweetener sorbitol, fruits with fructose can trigger diarrhea in some patients, and spicy foods. Carbonated beverages do not cause diarrhea, but they contain high levels of carbon dioxide, which can produce large amounts of gas when warmed in the stomach. For this reason, people with a gas problem should avoid or cut back on carbonated or "sparkling" drinks if they cause problems. Gas-producing foods include some fruits and vegetables, whole grains, and milk products. Because high-fat foods can increase bloating and discomfort, cutting back on these foods may help the stomach empty faster, allowing gases to move into the small intestine. Remember that the degree of stomach problems caused by certain foods varies from person to person. Effective dietary changes depend on learning through trial and error how much of any offending foods you can handle. Use your food diary to zoom in on trigger foods.

The Scoop on Portion Size

Because the size of a meal can increase muscle movement in the digestive tract and cause urgency to have a bowel movement, it is important to pay attention to both the nutritional makeup of your meal and as well its size. Check out the "servings per container" information listed on the Nutrition Facts on food packages. This can help you judge how much you are eating. When cooking at home, use a measuring cup and a food scale to gauge your usual food portions and compare these amounts to standard serving sizes on food labels for a week or so. Compare the suggested serving size listed on the label with the size of the portion you put on your plate before eating. This will help you get a feel for what one standard serving of a food looks compared to how much you normally eat. The label may say you are

Shrinking Portion Size by Tweaking Your Surroundings

Nutrition researchers have shown that one way of controlling portion size is by creating a home environment where you are less likely to eat large meals that can trigger or exacerbate IBS symptoms.

- *Eat meals at a table, not in front of the TV or computer.* Eating in front of the TV makes it hard to pay attention to your body's signals of fullness and may lead to eating large meals that can aggravate bowel problems.

- *Try to eat meals at regular intervals.* Skipping meals or leaving large gaps of time between meals may lead you to eat larger amounts of food the next time that you eat. This can aggravate IBS symptoms.

- *Eat when you're hungry.* If you eat when you're bored, bummed out, or because you don't have anything else to do, you are likely to eat larger meals that can trigger colonic contractions. Learn to recognize and control situational cues (like enticing aromas or a plate of homemade cookies on the kitchen counter) that cause us to feel hungry even when we aren't.

- *Eat slowly* so you give your brain the chance to register the message that your stomach is full.

- *Set your alarm early enough to eat breakfast.* People who eat breakfast are less likely to overeat later in the day.

- *When cooking large batches, freeze food that you will not serve right away.* This way, you will not be tempted to eat the whole batch before the food goes bad. And you will have ready-made food for another day. Freeze leftovers in amounts that you can use for a single serving or for a family meal another day.

consuming only 210 calories of macaroni but that is for ½ cup. If you eat a bowl full of pasta, you may be consuming two servings—and double the calories and fat (as well as other nutrients) in a standard serving. Chances are you'll be surprised to see how much you are eating.

Another way to learn healthy portion size is to use everyday items as a visual cue for standard single servings. The following examples can help you develop good "portion" sense:

- One serving of broccoli is the size of a light bulb.
- A 3-ounce serving of cooked meat is equal to the size of a deck of cards.
- 1 ½ ounces of low-fat or fat-free cheese equals 4 stacked dice.
- 1 tablespoon of mayo, oil, or dips equals a thumb tip.
- A serving of peanut butter (2 tablespoons) is the size of a golf ball.
- A serving of cereal or a potato (½ cup) is equivalent to a fist.
- 1 ounce serving of pretzels or snack food is a rounded handful.
- A serving size of cooked rice or pasta is the size of a baseball cut in half.

FOOD FOR THOUGHT

Because IBS can be so unpleasant and disruptive, many people desperately want to help themselves by finding a diet that rids them of their symptoms once and for all. There's no shortage of websites or books at your local bookstore featuring fad diets that promise IBS sufferers immediate relief. These diets often list "good" and "bad" foods, tout a "one size fits all" approach that ignores important differences among IBS patients, make dramatic statements ("100% guaranteed to eliminate IBS symptoms"), bait the reader with the promise of quick results wrapped around an intuitive but unproven medical-sounding rationale (such as flushing the gut of "toxic buildup"), and promote its legitimacy through paid celebrity endorsement or glowing patient testimonials not rigorous scientific research. In truth, there is no quick fix or miracle diet that will cure the full range of IBS symptoms. The most sensible and useful approach entails eating a healthful diet that provides adequate amounts of essential nutrients and calories while steering clear of specific triggers that aggravate your symptoms. Whether you are looking for a dietary approach as a primary treatment or as a way of boosting the value of medical or behavioral interventions, the information, tools, and strategies featured in this chapter should help you get the most out of dietary interventions and move you along the path toward better symptom self management.

THE ROLE OF MEDICATION IN CONTROLLING IBS

Jan, 33, is a sales representative for a medical device manufacturing company in southern Ontario, Canada. Her gastroenterologist diagnosed Jan with IBS-D three years ago shortly after she and her husband returned from their honeymoon in Mexico. She successfully completed the University at Buffalo IBS Treatment Program, where she learned a number of skills that can control the severity and frequency of symptoms. Nonetheless, she still struggles occasionally with episodes of diarrhea, particularly after eating fatty foods like her grandmother's tasty meat sauce. What works for Jan is keeping a small bottle of the antidiarrheal medication loperamide in her purse. She takes a pill before she goes out to eat or when she is heading off to a business meeting where she is unsure where a bathroom is located. This allows her to delay having a bowel movement for an hour or two until she finds a comfortable place to use the bathroom. This gives her added peace of mind when she is at work.

Although the treatment plan described in this book aims to give you a clinically proven drug-free option for taking control of even the most severe IBS symptoms, some people like Jan find that medication can be quite helpful for specific symptoms. This is understandable, because IBS is a complex problem for which there is no single treatment that works for all symptoms for everyone all the time. Some individuals may just prefer a pharmacologic approach. Others may find that learning skills to manage symptoms takes too much time to master, or that they're just not effective enough. Whether you may benefit from medication is a personal decision that you should make after talking with your doctor. The two of you should work together to find the treatment or combination of treatments that best fits your symptom profile, medical history, cost, and likely benefits, risks, and tolerance for side effects.

In this chapter, you'll learn basic information on the more common medications: their chemical and brand names, how they are supposed to work, the benefits you can realistically expect based on the current scientific evidence, and common side effects. The classes of medications commonly used to treat IBS include: laxatives and fiber supplements, antidiarrheals, antispasmodics, antidepressants, and two serotonin modifiers specifically developed for the multiple symptoms of IBS. You'll find an overview of the information presented in this chapter in the IBS Medications Chart on pages 226-227.

LAXATIVES

Laxatives are agents aimed at relieving constipation by regulating bowel function. There are several different types of laxatives, each of which is believed to work in different ways. These include fiber supplements and bulk-forming agents, osmotics, stimulants, and emollients. These categories reflect how they are believed to work.

Fiber Supplements and Bulk-Forming Agents

Dietary fiber and fiber supplements are types of laxatives that are considered to be bulk-forming agents because they absorb and retain fluid in the intestines, increasing the volume and softness of the stool. Because it is reasonably safe and inexpensive, fiber is a first-line treatment of choice by US physicians for the majority of IBS patients. Those with lumpy and hard stool are likely to improve the most from dietary fiber. Because dietary fiber absorbs water in the GI tract, it is also recommended for patients with loose, watery stool.

In the last chapter you learned about the possible benefits of increasing dietary fiber by eating more fiber-rich foods. Patients with milder forms of constipation find that dietary fiber can be quite effective. Dietary fiber works by absorbing liquid to form a larger stool. The presence of bulky stool stimulates the bowel muscles to contract. For this to happen, it may mean you often have to eat a lot of fiber. This can be hard to do without bringing on other unpleasant GI symptoms, such as gas or bloating.

One study found that one-third of patients on high-fiber diets experienced increased symptoms of bloating. In these cases, some patients try to increase the amount of dietary fiber by using fiber supplements. Fiber supplements come in a concentrated form of natural fiber (wheat bran, corn fiber) or dry tablets and are available over-the-counter at drug stores, supermarkets, or health food shops. They are usually made from the walls of plant seeds. When mixed with water and consumed, the fiber in the supplement swells, making your stool softer and bigger. Popular fiber supplements include psyllium seed husks (Metamucil, ispaghula husk, Fiberall), calcium polycarbophil (Fiber Con) or methylcellulose (Citrucel). To work effectively, fiber supplements should be taken with lots of water (at least one to two glasses per dose) to prevent your bowels from getting blocked. Patients who can't consume an adequate amount of water (half a gallon a day) are discouraged from starting a high-fiber diet. It is not recommended that fiber supplements be taken just before going to bed.

While high-fiber diets and fiber supplements appear to improve constipation in some patients, there is conflicting evidence as to whether they provide any more global relief from IBS symptoms than a placebo treatment (sugar pill). Moreover, any relief they may provide usually occurs slowly (between 12 and 72 hours after ingestion), making it a poor option for rapid relief of symptom flare-ups. Dietary fiber may worsen pain, diarrhea, and bloating, and has no established benefit for the abdominal pain of IBS.

If symptoms don't respond to the addition of fiber, patients may be prescribed one of the other types of laxatives.

Osmotics

Osmotic laxatives contain chemical substances that draw more water into the bowel so that less fluid is absorbed into the bloodstream. This process, called osmosis, bulks up the size of the stool. Because osmotic laxatives increase the amount of water in the colon, it's important to drink lots of water (up to half a gallon of water a day). Osmotic laxatives, which may take a few days to take effect, are available as powders, liquids, or enemas. Examples of osmotic laxatives include:

- Magnesium citrate (Citroma)
- Magnesium hydroxide (Philips Milk of Magnesia)
- Lactulose (Acilac, Cephulac, Cholac, Chronulac)
- Polyethylene (Miralax)

While magnesium-based laxatives are generally safe and well tolerated, lactulose can cause abdominal cramping, gas, bloating, and diarrhea, making it a poor option for long-term use. Because osmotic laxatives speed the flow of fluids through the GI tract, they can interfere with absorption of other drugs. Generally speaking, there is limited scientific evidence supporting the use of osmotic laxatives for IBS. Nonetheless, osmotic laxatives are occasionally recommended, particularly for patients who have not responded to fiber and bulking agents. Some constipated patients treated with osmotic laxatives develop diarrhea.

Stimulant Laxatives

Patients who don't respond to osmotic laxatives may be prescribed stimulant laxatives, which are available as tablets or suppositories. Stimulant laxatives include:

- Senna (Senokot)
- Bisacodyl (Dulcolax, Correctol)

These laxatives increase water and salt secretion into the colon, stimulating the nerve endings in the intestinal lining to trigger contractions that move the stool mass along the GI tract. They work more quickly (within 8 to 12 hours) than osmotic laxatives or fiber supplements, and are therefore a good match for patients needing rapid relief for acute attacks. However, there haven't been any controlled medical studies confirming their usefulness for IBS patients. For this reason, stimulant laxatives are typically not recommended for IBS.

Because of the way they work, stimulant laxatives can cause cramping, bloating, dehydration (not enough water in the body), and an imbalance in naturally ocuring minerals (electrolytes) such as potassium. In rare cases, overuse of stimulant laxatives reportedly causes the digestive system to become too reliant on laxatives to carry out normal bowel functions (this is called *lazy bowel syndrome*). Because they can be habit forming, long-term use of stimulant laxatives is typically discouraged. This makes them a poor option for the constipated IBS patient looking for a long-term option.

Emollients

Another type of laxative are the emollients, which boost the amount of water in the stool, thus lubricating the stool so that it is softer and easier to pass. Mineral oil suppositories and stool softeners fall into this category.

Mineral oil suppositories coat the bowel and the stool with a water-proof film; these emollients retain moisture in the stool and ease the passage of bowel movements. Mineral oil has not been found to change bowel function. The most common side effect among patients who use mineral oil is that the suppository leaks into their underwear. Additional side effects include nausea, skin rash, diarrhea, and cramping.

Stool softeners are believed to work by increasing the amount of fluid in the stool. One example is docusate (Colace), which is available as an over-the-counter product. These laxatives soften hard stool and allow one to pass a bowel movement without straining. However, they don't stimulate a bowel movement or reduce constipation. The main side effects of docusate are bitter taste, throat irritation, and nausea for patients who use the syrup and liquid forms. Because side effects are generally infrequent and not severe, these laxatives are regarded as safer than other types. Docusate is an emulsifying agent that increases the absorption of mineral oil, so for that reason these two emollients should not be used in combination.

ANTIDIARRHEALS

Antidiarrheal medications are a mainstay of treating diarrhea and are commonly prescribed for IBS patients whose primary symptoms include diarrhea. These drugs aim to keep dehydration in check and slow the rate of movement of food through the gut so that more fluid is absorbed. Two common antidiarrheals are loperamide (Imodium) and diphenoxylate (Lomotil). Neither agent is intended for long-term use. Instead, they are best used preventively to minimize the likelihood of mild, short-lived diarrhea attacks that interfere with work or social occasions.

Loperamide

In the United States, loperamide is available in liquid and tablet form as an over-the-counter medication and is believed to ease diarrhea by increasing the absorption of water in the GI tract and slowing down intestinal motility. This reduces the time it takes material to move through the digestive system, resulting in a decrease in stool frequency and urgency and improves stool consistency. While loperamide is a reasonably effective drug for diarrhea, its ability to relieve the multiple symptoms (such as pain or bloating) that characterize IBS is unproven. It's possible that antidiarrheals have psychological benefits as well as physical ones. Taking an antidiarrheal as a preventive measure before taking a trip or going out for an important event (giving a speech, attending a meeting or sporting event) can dampen anxiety that may otherwise aggravate bowel symptoms.

Common side effects of loperamide include constipation, abdominal cramps, drowsiness, dizziness, dry mouth, fatigue, and nausea, although most patients tolerate loperamide reasonably well. Some patients find that if they split their daily dose into smaller doses, they experience less stomach cramping at night.

Diphenoxylate

Diphenoxylate is available in prescription form under the brand name of Lomotil. It combines two agents: diphenoxylate and atropine. While diphenoxylate can slow down intestinal contractions and therefore improve diarrhea, it is an opiate and therefore potentially habit forming. For this reason, small amounts of atropine are added so that individuals experience undesirable side effects such as dry mouth, nausea, and weakness if they use diphenoxylate in high dosages and/or over a long period of time for recreational purposes. Side effects of diphenoxylate include abdominal pain, dizziness, drowsiness, dry mouth, and headache. These side effects typically diminish as your body adjusts to the medication

*

Of the two antidiarrheals, physicians often prefer loperamide over diphenoxylate because loperamide has a low potential for addiction. Loperamide's effects last longer and are less likely to cause abdominal pain and bloating than diphenoxylate. Because antidiarrheals can improve muscle tone around the anus, there is some evidence that they can reduce fecal incontinence (inability to control bowel movements).

ANTISPASMODICS

Many doctors prescribe antispasmodics for patients whose gut pain doesn't respond to simple lifestyle and dietary changes (such as increasing dietary fiber). These medications are believed to reduce pain and bloating by relaxing the muscle in the wall of the gut and relieving muscle spasms. While scientific evidence has largely rejected the notion that IBS symptoms are caused strictly by bowel spasms (see the first chapter of the book), these studies have had little impact on the widespread use of antispasmodics. Antispasmodics remain one of the world's most prescribed IBS drugs for pain. For people whose gut pain begins after eating (postprandial pain), some people find that taking an antispasmodic right before a meal can help ward off symptoms. Some people take an antispasmodic medication for a couple of weeks to take the edge off acute pain flare up.

There are three primary types of antispasmodics—anticholinergics, peppermint oil, and direct muscle relaxants (not available in the US).

Anticholinergics

Anticholinergic agents block the effect of acetylcholine, a brain chemical that causes smooth muscles in the GI tract (and other parts of the body) to contract. The belief is that by relaxing the muscles of the GI tract, anticholinergic antispasmodics decrease muscle spasms and the discomfort and urgency that comes with having a bowel movement. Anticholinergic drugs used to treat IBS include:

- Dicyclomine (Bentyl)
- Hyoscyamine (Levsin)
- Chlordiazepoxide combined with clinidium (Librax)

Antispasmodics are best used about 30 minutes before meals to prevent sudden painful flare-ups. While anticholinergic agents are some of the most commonly prescribed medications for IBS, there is inconclusive evidence that they are better than placebo in reducing pain and constipation. Anticholinergic antispasmodics can have side effects, including headache, blurred vision, constipation, lightheadedness, urination problems, dizziness, nasal stuffiness, rash, and dry mouth. The unpleasantness of these side effects restricts their use, particularly over the long term. Because the side effects of antispasmodics include constipation, they are sometimes recommended for IBS patients whose primary complaint is diarrhea.

Peppermint Oil

A second class of antispasmodics is peppermint oil. Peppermint oil directly relaxes bowel muscles by blocking the entry of calcium into the muscle cells. Because an influx of calcium is believed to trigger muscle contractions, agents such as peppermint oil that block calcium are believed to keep strong muscle contractions "turned off." Only a handful of studies have formally studied the usefulness of peppermint oil for the treatment of IBS. The results suggest that peppermint oil may be a bit more effective than placebo in treating specific IBS symptoms (particularly gas, cramping, and discomfort). Coated peppermint tablets (Elanco Lakcaps) can reduce the side effects of nausea and heartburn by delaying the oil from dissolving in the stomach before reaching the small intestine. Coated capsules may cause a burning sensation in the anus. Other side effects of peppermint oil include upset stomach, blurred vision, and heartburn.

Direct Smooth Muscle Relaxants

In Canada, Australia, and Europe, IBS patients have access to another class of antispasmodics called direct smooth muscle relaxants. These drugs work by relaxing the smooth muscles of the gut. Examples of direct muscle relaxants include mebeverine (Duspatalin, Colofac), pinaverium (Dicetal), and trimebutine (Modulon). Randomized studies show direct muscle relaxants to be more effective than placebo in improving global ratings of IBS symptoms and reducing abdominal pain, although the studies were not of the best quality. Side effects of direct muscle relaxants, while rare, include allergic reactions such as inflamed or reddened skin, itchy skin, rashes or severe swelling of lips, face, or tongue.

ANTIDEPRESSANTS

Your doctor may prescribe certain antidepressants to treat various aspects of IBS if simple lifestyle changes or dietary treatments don't work. Antidepressants alter the balance of some brain chemical messengers (neurotransmitters such as serotonin and norepinephrine) that help neighboring nerve cells communicate with each other. Antidepressants were initially developed to treat depression, but it was discovered that they have pain-reducing properties when given at lower dosages than used to treat depression (provided there is no coexisting depression). This is because some neurotransmitters help block pain signals delivered to the spinal cord from nerve endings. The two classes of antidepressants commonly used for IBS are tricyclic antidepressants (TCAs) and the selective serotonin reuptake inhibitors (SSRIs).

Tricyclic Antidepressants

One group of drugs that is effective at relieving pain is the family of antidepressants called the tricyclics or TCAs. The word "tricyclic" refers to their three-ringed chemical structure. Here's how tricyclics are believed to work. After nerve endings release serotonin, they quickly suck it up again. TCA antidepressants such as amitriptyline (Elavil), imipramine (Tofranil), and trazodone (Desyrel) block the removal of neurotransmitters so that they stay in the gaps between nerve cells. This prolongs the neurotransmitters' effect so they continue to suppress the transmission of pain signals to the brain. The pain-relieving effects of TCAs are independent of their effects on mood. So don't be alarmed if your doctor recommends that you give an antidepressant a try. It doesn't necessarily mean you're depressed, or that your physical symptoms are in your head! It is important to remember that TCAs do not immediately relieve pain. It may take several weeks before the pain-reducing effects are felt. Even then, patients taking TCAs can realistically expect a modest improvement in abdominal pain.

Of course, if you're struggling with marked feelings of depression or anxiety that don't go away, there's nothing wrong with getting help, and antidepressants are a clinically proven method that may help. However, the effectiveness of TCAs for nonpainful IBS bowel symptoms (e.g., bloating, diarrhea, constipation) is inconclusive. A recent summary of studies suggests that less than a third of IBS patients treated with TCAs responded well, although another study painted a more favorable picture of the benefits of TCAs, particularly in patients with diarrhea and pain. If your doctor does prescribe a TCA for IBS symptoms, you should know it isn't likely to provide overall relief from the full range of IBS symptoms, and it can cause side effects.

The most common side effects of TCAs include sedation, dry mouth, temporary lightheadedness, urinary retention, weight gain, rapid heartbeat, low blood pressure, and constipation. Of course, some side effects (such as constipation, sedation) may help you if your primary bowel problem is diarrhea or if you have trouble sleeping. Because of their sedating effects, TCAs are often prescribed at bedtime for patients with sleep problems. TCAs can cause disturbance in heart rhythm, which creates potential problems for patients with heart disease. Elderly patients treated with TCAs may experience mental confusion, balance problems, or delirium.

The side effects of TCAs are unpleasant but not typically dangerous. Experiencing side effects doesn't mean that the medication is harming your body. Indeed, side effects mean that the medication is having a desired chemical effect on your body. Patients often find the side effects worse during the first few weeks as their body adjusts to a new medication. Side effects may occur before antidepressant activity does. Side effects usually diminish after a few weeks. Among tricyclic antidepressants, experts believe that desipramine (Norpamin) and nortriptyline (Pamelor) have fewer side effects than Elavil and imipramine (Tofranil). Because IBS is more common among females, it is important to know that women have a harder time tolerating side effects of imipramine. While many patients tolerate side effects over time, others find them so unpleasant that they stop taking them, or don't take a sufficient dose of the medicine to get its full benefit. Antidepressant medications in general must be taken regularly for three to four weeks (in some cases as many as eight weeks) before experiencing improvement. Some patients find them easier to tolerate by beginning with a low dose, taking the dose a few hours before bedtime, and slowly increasing the dose under the guidance of a physician over the first few weeks when side effects are strongest and most difficult to bear.

TCAs are generally easy to discontinue, less expensive, and no less effective than the newer antidepressants described below. Because TCAs are not effective over the long haul unless you continue to take them, many patients find them costly and inconvenient. Patients often are tempted to stop taking tryicyclics (and other antidepressants) too soon. They may feel better and believe the medication is no longer needed. It is important to keep taking the medication for at least four to nine months to prevent a return of symptoms.

Selective Serotonin Reuptake Inhibitors

Another class of newer antidepressants is the selective serotonin reuptake inhibitors (SSRIs). These drugs block serotonin receptors from reabsorbing serotonin after it is released in the gap between nerve cells in the brain. By making serotonin usable in the brain, SSRIs boost serotonin levels, which some scientists link to depression and other psychiatric disorders. Examples of SSRIs include:

- Paroxetine (Paxil)
- Sertraline (Zoloft)
- Fluoxetine (Prozac)
- Citalopram (Celexa)

SSRIs can improve feelings of anxiety or depression, but their benefits for IBS symptoms like pain, diarrhea, or constipation are unproven. One recent small study showed that the SSRI citalopram (Celexa) improves general well being and reduces the number of days with abdominal pain relief in some patients. However, there was only a modest effect on stool patterns. Because of their inconsistent impact on IBS symptoms, SSRIs are typically reserved for patients with marked feelings of anxiety or depression. Because SSRIs just act on serotonin receptors, they have fewer and weaker side effects than TCAs, which influence other neurotransmitters. SSRIs are less likely to be discontinued because of side effects.

The most commonly reported side effects of SSRIs are mild headache, daytime drowsiness, sleep disturbance, nausea, and loss of sexual desire. As with all medications, not everyone treated with SSRIs experiences side effects, which can vary considerably from person to person. Like TCAs, the side effects of SSRIs are most annoying and worrisome during the first few months, as the body adjusts to the chemical effects of the drug. Side effects usually diminish within two to three weeks of starting a prescription. Most SSRIs are available in a single daily dose, and they are less likely to interact negatively with other medications and less dangerous if taken as an overdose. As with TCAs, patients treated with SSRIs may not begin to experience an improvement in symptoms for up to four to six weeks after starting treatment. While SSRIs are not addictive (don't cause craving or tolerance), some patients experience symptoms when discontinuing them, missing doses, or reducing the dose. Sudden discontinuation of SSRIs can cause temporary withdrawal symptoms such as flulike symptoms (headache, diarrhea, nausea, vomiting, chills, dizziness, fatigue), insomnia, balance problems, and sensitivity to outside stimuli. These symptoms— called discontinuation syndrome—are mild, typically last one to two weeks, and end when medication is restarted. Discontinuation syndrome occurs with medications in other families of antidepressants as well but is more common in the SSRI family, particularly those like (citalopram) Celexa or Paxil (paroxetine) that remain in the bloodstream longer (shorter half life). To minimize the risk of these symptoms, it is important to gradually decrease medication under the supervision of your treating physician so that your body has time to adjust. As with TCAs, once you discontinue SSRIs the risks that symptoms are likely to return is about as high as before you began taking the drug.

SEROTONIN MODIFIERS

Serotonin not only influences our moods but also helps the digestive system functional normally. While serotonin is found in both the brain and gut, 95 percent of the body's serotonin is located in the gut! The serotonin housed there is believed to play an important role in the control of abdominal pain perception, contraction of gut muscles, and release of fluids into the GI tract. Many scientists believe that IBS is related to the way the digestive system reacts to changes in gut serotonin. Too much serotonin can cause diarrhea. Too little serotonin creates the opposite effect of constipation. For these reasons, two of the newest IBS drugs—alosetron (Lotronex) and tegaserod (Zelnorm)—were specifically designed to zero in on specific serotonin receptors in the GI tract that increase the sensation of pain and affect bowel function. By targeting multiple GI symptoms (pain, bloating, bowel problems), both alosetron and tegaserod have advantages over older drugs that target single symptoms of IBS. Both alosetron and tegaserod are more expensive than other drugs used to treat IBS. It is estimated that these drugs cost about $5–6 per dose and require patients to take them twice a day. By comparison, the common diarrhea medicine loperamide costs about 60 cents per dose.

Alosetron (Lotronex)

Alosetron is used to treat women with IBS who have severe diarrhea as their main symptom (diarrhea-predominant IBS). Clinical trials show that it helps about one out of seven patients. Alosetron's benefits include improved pain/discomfort, urgency, stool frequency, and increased stool consistency in women with IBS. By blocking the action of serotonin receptors in the wall of the gut, alosetron is believed to normalize bowel activity by slowing down the movement of waste through the colon, controlling how much pain is perceived, and decreasing release of fluid into the intestines. Patients treated with alosetron report more satisfactory relief from pain/discomfort, firmer stool, and significantly fewer bowel movements than treated patients treated with placebo. The value of these findings is weakened by the fact that in at least 30 percent of people using alosetron and other IBS drugs, a dummy drug with no direct chemical effects (placebo) works just as well. In other words, the psychological benefit of being administered a pill that's meant to help you has real physical benefit. The benefits of alosetron on bowel symptoms appear to diminish quickly when it is discontinued, suggesting that it is best for short-term use. Alosetron hasn't been shown to help men with IBS or women whose primary symptom is constipation.

Common side effects of alosetron include constipation that begins during the first month of treatment and goes away on its own or after treatment is interrupted. Within a year of its release, the Food and Drug Administration received a limited number of reports of severe constipation and a condition called ischemic colitis, which is caused by lack of blood flow to the bowel. Major side effects occurred in 1 out of every 250 patients treated with alosetron, and five deaths were tied to its use as well. Even though these risks were relatively rare, their seriousness prompted the withdrawal of alosetron from the market in 2000. To meet public demand, it was reapproved by the FDA two years later and today can be prescribed by specially certified physicians under a rigorous monitoring plan that requires patients to sign a special consent before using the drug. Because of potential side effects, alosetron is available for female patients with severe diarrhea-prominent IBS (not for those with primary bowel problems of constipation or constipation alternating with diarrhea) who have not responded to other treatments.

Tegaserod (Zelnorm)

While alosetron slows the movement of stool by blocking specific serotonin receptors, tegaserod stimulates other receptors. This action reduces sensitivity to gut stimulation, speeds up muscle contractions in the bowel that push stool through the colon, and increases production of fluid in the bowels. These changes are believed to decrease constipation and pain associated with IBS. In clinical studies using a comparison group of constipation-predominant IBS patients taking a placebo (dummy) treatment, patients rated the effectiveness of tegaserod as higher than placebo. Tegaserod appears most effective in providing an overall sense of improvement for symptoms associated with constipation-predominant IBS (pain, bloating, constipation). Patients treated with tegaserod have more bowel movements and fewer days without bowel movements Whether Tegaserod consistently improves individual IBS symptoms such as pain, stool consistency, straining and bloating is unclear. Treatment benefits occur most noticeably during the first month of treatment. Whether tegaserod is safe and effective for men with constipation-predominant IBS is not proven. Like alosetron, patients treated with tegaserod relapse when they stop taking the medication. There is some reason to believe that the relief patients receive from tegaserod diminishes somewhat after the first month of treatment. For this reason, tegaserod is typically recommended for short-term use.

Common side effects occur infrequently, but include headache, abdominal pain, diarrhea, nausea, and gas. In March, 2007, the manufacturer of tegaserod (Novartis Pharmaceuticals) voluntarily suspended marketing and sales of this drug at the request of the FDA because of a small but statistically significant number of serious cardiovascular adverse events (angina, myocardial infarctions, and strokes) in patients who had undergone clinical trials. It is unclear whether tegaserod will be reintroduced to the market. It is possible that Novartis will reintroduce the drug if a population of patients can be identified in which the benefits of the drug are viewed as clearly outweighing the risks.

*

The IBS Medications Chart on pages 226-227 condenses all the information in this chapter into a concise format that may be helpful as you consider the many options available.

This chapter has given you basic information about the types of medications prescribed for IBS, their side effects, and their potential value. As you can see, there is no single "wonder drug" or class of medication that works for the full range of IBS symptoms. A surprising number of commonly prescribed medications fare no better than placebo in relieving symptoms. Each medication targets specific symptoms and has its pluses and minuses. Most are designed either for short-term use (such as the antidiarrheals), or require prolonged use (such as the antidepressants) to maintain benefit. If you are looking for a medical option either as a main treatment or an addition to other therapies, speak to your doctor about the benefits and side effects you're likely to experience and how the prescribed medication will realistically impact your specific IBS symptoms.

IBS Medications Chart

LAXATIVES

Generic Name (Brand Name)	Target Symptom(s)	Common Side Effects
Fiber Supplements/Bulking Agents Psyllium (*Metamucil*) Polycarbophil (*FiberCon*) Methylcellulose (*Citrucel*)	•constipation •diarrhea (occasionally)	•bloating •pain •gas
Osmotic Laxatives Magnesium citrate (*Citroma*) Lactulose (*Acilac, Cephulac,* *Cholac, Chronulac*) Polyethylene glycol (*MiraLax*) Magnesium hydroxide (*Milk of Magnesia*)	•constipation	•bloating •gas •nausea •abdominal cramping
Stimulant Laxatives Senna (*Senokot, ExLax*) Bisacodyl (*Dulcolax, Correctol*)	•constipation	•intestinal cramps •bloating •fluid loss •electrolyte imbalance •diarrhea
Emollient Laxatives Mineral oil (*Fleet mineral oil*) Docusate (*Colace*)	•constipation	•bitter taste •nausea •suppository leaks

ANTIDIARRHEALS

Generic Name (Brand Name)	Target Symptom(s)	Common Side Effects
Loperamide (*Imodium*)	•diarrhea •urgency	•abdominal pain •constipation •drowsiness •dizziness •dry mouth •fatigue •nausea •vomiting
Dipenoxylate atropine (*Lomotil*)	•diarrhea	•diarrhea •pain •dizziness •drowsiness •dry mouth •headache •nausea •vomiting •rash

IBS Medications Chart

ANTISPASMODICS

Generic Name (Brand Name)	Target Symptom(s)	Common Side Effects
Anticholinergics Dicyclimone (Bentyl) Hyoscyamine (Levsin) Chlordiazepoxide combined with clinidium (Librax)	•intestinal cramps •pain after meals	•headache •dizziness •blurred vision •rash/ itching •constipation •dry mouth •confusion •difficult urinating
Peppermint oil (Elanco Lakcaps)	•intestinal cramps	•heartburn •blurred vision •upset stomach •burning sensation around the anus
Direct Smooth Muscle Relaxants *Mebeverine (Duspatalin, Colofac), *Pinaverium (Dicetal) *Trimebutine (Modulon) _{*not available in U.S.}	•intestinal cramps	•inflamed or reddened skin, •itchy skin, •swelling of lips, face or tongue

ANTIDEPRESSANTS

Generic Name (Brand Name)	Target Symptom(s)	Common Side Effects

Tricyclics (TCAs)
Amitriptyline (Elavil)
Imipramine (Tofranil)
Trazode (Desyrel)
Desipramine (Norpamin)
Nortriptyline (Pamelor)
Doxepin (Sinequan)
	•coexisting anxiety,
	  depression
	•abdominal pain
	•diarrhea
	•nausea
		•drowsiness
		•increased appetite
		•dizziness
		•difficult urinating
		•weight gain
		•disturbance of
		  heart rhythm
		•low blood pressure
		•constipation
		•dry mouth
		•blurred vision

Selective Serotonin Reuptake Inhibitors (SSRIs) Paroxetine (Paxil) Sertraline (Zoloft) Fluoxetine (Prozac) Citalopram (Celexa) Mirtazipine (Remeron)	•coexisting anxiety, depression	•diarrhea or constipation •headache •drowsiness/ fatigue •weight gain •sleep disturbance •nausea •reduced sexual desire •dizziness

SEROTONIN MODIFIERS

Generic Name (Brand Name)	Target Symptom(s)	Common Side Effects
Alosetron (Lotronex)	•diarrhea •abdominal pain	•constipation
Tegaserod (Zelnorm) _{NOTE: As of March 2007 tegaserod was withdrawn from the market (see page 224).}	•constipation •abdominal pain •bloating	•headache •abdominal pain •diarrhea

APPENDIX

GLOSSARY

abdomen The large cavity between the chest and the pelvis containing the stomach, small intestine, colon (large bowel), liver, gallbladder, and spleen.

acute A disorder that is sudden and lasts only a short period of time (typically 3-6 months).

adrenaline A chemical in the body that relaxes the muscles and decreases blood flow to the stomach and intestines. Also called epinephrine.

alarm symptoms A characteristic of a serious GI disease caused by damage to the gut. Alarm symptoms include (but are not limited to) fever, unintentional weight loss, and bloody stool. These symptoms are not characteristics of irritable bowel syndrome. Also called red flags.

allergy A condition in which the body is not able to tolerate certain foods, animals, plants, or other substances.

anemia A condition in which the number of red blood cells is less than normal, resulting in less oxygen being carried to the body's cells.

antibodies A molecule tailor made by the immune system to lock onto and destroy specific foreign substances as bacteria and viruses.

anticholinergics Medicines that calm muscle spasms in the intestine. Examples include dicyclomine (Bentyl) and hyoscyamine (Levsin).

antidiarrheals Medicines that help control diarrhea. An example is loperamide (Imodium).

antispasmodics Medicines that help reduce or stop muscle spasms in the intestines. Examples are dicyclomine (Bentyl) and atropine (Donnatal). Used to treat abdominal pain.

anus The opening of the digestive tract through which feces (bowel movements) are discharged.

appendicitis An inflammation of the appendix caused by infection, scarring, or blockage.

appendix A 4-inch pouch attached to the first part of the large intestine (cecum). No one knows what function the appendix has, if any.

autoantibodies Antibodies that attack the body itself.

autonomic nervous system The part of the nervous system that controls muscles of internal organs (such as the heart, blood vessels, lungs, stomach, and intestines) and glands (such as salivary glands and sweat glands). One part of the ANS helps the body rest, relax, and digest food and another part helps a person fight or take flight in an emergency. Also called involuntary nervous system.

bacteria A large group of single-cell microorganisms. Some cause infections and disease in animals and humans.

bacterial overgrowth A condition that involves large numbers of bacteria growing in the small intestine.

barium A silver-white metallic compound that helps to show the image of the lower gastrointestinal tract on an X-ray.

barium enema A diagnostic procedure in which X-rays are taken after barium sulfate is introduced into the patient by enema. The barium sulfate helps to outline the colon and rectum so that they appear on X-rays.

barium meal A diagnostic procedure in which X-rays are taken after the patient swallows barium sulfate. The barium sulfate helps to outline the esophagus, stomach and duodenum so that they appear on X-rays. Also called barium swallow.

biopsy A test that involves collecting small pieces of tissue, usually through a needle, for examination under a microscope.

bloating Fullness or swelling in the abdomen that often occurs after meals.

bowel Another word for the small and large intestine.

bowel movement Body wastes passed through the rectum and anus.

bulking agents Laxatives that make bowel movements soft and easy to pass. Common laxatives include bran and other bulking agents such as psyllium.

celiac disease The inability to digest and absorb gluten, the protein found in wheat. Undigested gluten causes damage to the lining of the small intestine, which prevents absorption of nutrients from other foods. Also called celiac sprue, gluten intolerance, and nontropical sprue.

cholecystokinin (CCK) A hormone released by the intestine in response to food; CCK causes the gallbladder and the colon to contract and release stored bile.

chronic Refers to disorders lasting a long duration or that frequently recur over a long period.

colitis Inflammation of the colon.

colon The last portion of your digestive tract, or GI tract. Also known as the large bowel or large intestine.

colonoscope A flexible tube with a light on the end used to view the entire colon.

colonoscopy A diagnostic test that permits a doctor to look inside the entire large intestine for inflamed tissue, abnormal growths, and ulcers. It is most often used to look for early signs of cancer in the colon and rectum. It is also used to look for causes of unexplained changes in bowel habits and to evaluate symptoms like abdominal pain, rectal bleeding, and weight loss.

colorectal cancer Cancer that occurs in the colon (large intestine) or the rectum (the end of the large intestine). Medical researchers have found no relationship between having IBS and the risk of developing colorectal or any other form of cancer.

complete blood count (CBC) A laboratory test performed on a sample of blood, which measures the percentage of red blood cells present.

computerized tomography (CT or CAT) scan A painless diagnostic procedure in which the X-ray source rotates around the patient so that an x-ray beam is sent through the patient from may different angles. The X-rays is read by a computer which constructs three-dimensional images of the body.

constipation A condition in which the stool becomes hard and dry. A person who is constipated usually has fewer than three bowel movements in a week. Bowel movements may be painful, infrequent and /or difficult to pass.

Crohn's disease A type of inflammatory bowel disease that causes severe inflammation in the gastrointestinal tract. It usually affects the lower small intestine (ileum) or the colon, but it can affect the entire gastrointestinal tract. See also Inflammatory Bowel Disease (IBD).

dehydration A condition caused by loss of too much water from the body. Dehydration can be caused by severe diarrhea or vomiting.

diagnostic imaging The use of X-ray or ultrasound pictures of the body organs to make diagnoses.

diaphragm The muscle wall between the chest and the abdomen. It is the major muscle that the body uses for breathing.

diarrhea Frequent, loose, and watery bowel movements. Common causes include gastrointestinal infections, irritable bowel syndrome, medicines, and malabsorption.

dietary fiber Fiber is the part of foods such as fruits, vegetables, legumes, and whole grains that cannot be digested. Because fiber resists digestion in the gastrointestinal tract, it

accounts for a significant portion of the solid matter in bowel movements.

digestion The process the body uses to break down food into simple substances that are capable of being absorbed by the intestines for energy, growth, and cell repair.

digestive system The organs in the body that break down and absorb food. Organs that make up the digestive system are the mouth, esophagus, stomach, small intestine, large intestine, rectum, and anus.

digestive tract See **gastrointestinal (GI) tract.**

digital rectal exam An exam were a doctor uses a gloved hand to check the rectum to see if it feels normal.

discontinuation syndrome Withdrawal symptoms that may occur when a particular medication is abruptly stopped (flulike symptoms, insomnia, balance problems, and sensitivity to outside stimuli).

distention A visible increase in the waistline; often occurring after meals.

diuretic A substance that causes an increased flow of urine.

diverticulitis A condition in which diverticula become inflamed

diverticulosis A condition in which small sacs (diverticula) form in the wall of the colon. This condition is common among older people.

diverticulum/diverticula A small sac(s) that forms on the wall of a hollow organ (usually the colon).

duodenum The first part of the small intestine.

dyspepsia Another name for indigestion.

endometriosis A disease in which tissue that normally lines the uterus grows in other areas of the body, most commonly in the pelvic region. This irregular growth causes pain, irregular bleeding, and could lead to infertility.

endoscope A small, flexible tube-like instrument, with a light on the end of it consisting of thousands of tiny glass fibers, that allows a doctor to see into the esophagus, stomach, duodenum, and colon. An endoscope also allows a doctor to perform biopsies, take color photographs, and perform certain medical procedures that would otherwise require surgery.

endoscopic retrograde cholangiopancreatography (ERCP) A diagnostic examination performed by a physician through an endoscope. A catheter is placed through the endoscope into the opening where the bile ducts and pancreas enter the duodenum and dye is injected. An X-ray is taken during the injection to permit the doctor to see the system of ducts.

endoscopy A procedure in which an endoscope is used.

enteritis Inflammation of the small intestine.

enzyme A protein that speeds up certain chemical processes. In the intestine, enzymes are needed to break down many foods into simpler substances so that they can be absorbed.

epinephrine A naturally occurring hormone transmitted across the gaps or synapses between neurons. Also called adrenaline, epinephrine plays an important role in activating the fight-or-flight response to stress.

erythrocyte sedimentation rate A test that measures the settling of red blood cells during a one hour period. The rate of settling is an indication of the level of inflammation present.

esophagitis Inflammation of the esophagus.

esophagus The organ that connects the mouth with the stomach.

estrogen A female reproductive hormone produced by the ovaries (found in smaller quantities in men) that is responsible for regulating a women's menstrual cycle and reproductive health

euphoria A feeling of elation or well-being that can be produced by recreational use of specific medications.

fecal incontinence The inability to control bowel movements.

feces Solid body wastes, passed as bowel movements. See also **stool**.

fiber A substance in foods that come from plants but is not digested by humans. Fiber helps bowel function by keeping stool soft so that it moves smoothly through the colon.

fight-or-flight response The body's natural reaction to an emergency. The body systems that are useful for facing a physically dangerous threat ("fight") or fleeing danger ("flight") are stimulated: Blood flow is increased to the muscles, heart rate, respiration, and blood pressure increase. As a tradeoff, energy is decreased to other ongoing body functions that are not immediately critical to survival (e.g., digestion, the body's immunity, ovulation).

fissure A deep crack.

fistula An abnormal hollow connection between two internal organs or between an internal organ and the outside body.

flatulence The passage of gas through the rectum, a normal occurrence, but troublesome if the frequency or volume is excessive or if the sound or odor is offensive.

functional Refers to how something works. A functional GI disorder is a medical disorder whose problem involves how the gut works.

functional disorders Disorders such as irritable bowel syndrome that are caused by faulty neural connections between the brain and gut. Common symptoms include pain, constipation, and diarrhea that that are not explained by physical disease or damage to the GI tract. Emotional stress can aggravate but does not cause functional disorders.

gallbladder A sac located beneath the liver that stores bile, a liquid used to help the body digest fats.

gas Air that comes from normal breakdown of food. The gases are passed out of the body through the rectum (flatus) or mouth (burp).

gastric juices Liquids produced in the stomach to aid digestion and kill bacteria.

gastritis Inflammation of the lining of the stomach.

gastroenterologist A doctor who specializes in treating diseases and disorders of the digestive system.

gastrointestinal (GI) Refers to the esophagus, stomach, small intestine, large intestine or colon, rectum, or anus.

gastrointestinal (GI) tract Includes the esophagus, stomach, small intestine, large intestine or colon, rectum, and anus. Also called alimentary canal or digestive tract.

GI See **gastrointestinal.**

gluten A protein found in wheat and some other grains. When people with celiac disease eat foods containing gluten, their immune system responds by damaging the small intestine.

gut See **intestines.**

hemoglobin The part of the red blood cell that binds to oxygen and carries it from the lungs to the tissues.

hemorrhoids Dilation of the veins in the anal area. The problems associated with hemorrhoids occur when these veins become enlarged, prolapsed, or become plugged or inflamed.

hereditary A term used to describe conditions that are passed genetically from parents to children.

hormone A substance in the body that regulates certain organs.

Hormones such as gastrin help in breaking down food. Some hormones come from cells in the stomach and small intestine.

hydrogen breath test Measures the amount of hydrogen present in a person's breath. Raised levels of hydrogen indicate lactose intolerance.

hyperthyroidism Excessive levels of thyroid hormones in the blood circulation. Signs and symptoms include weight loss, anxiety, palpitations, and heat intolerance.

hypothyroidism Low levels of thyroid hormones in the blood circulation. Signs and symptoms include weakness, fatigue, cold intolerance, constipation, and weight gain.

immune system The system that protects the body from viruses, bacteria, or any other foreign substances.

indigestion A term used to indicate any disruption in the digestive process. Symptoms commonly include heartburn, nausea, bloating, and gas. Doctors often call it dyspepsia.

infection Occurs when the body can't protect itself against microorganisms such as bacteria, viruses, or fungi.

infectious diarrhea (traveler's diarrhea) A diarrheal illness caused by an infectious agent: bacterial, viral, or protozoan.

inflammation A condition in which the body is trying to respond to localized injury or destruction of tissues. All or some of these signs are present: redness, heat, swelling, pain, and loss of function.

inflammatory bowel disease (IBD) Long-lasting problems that cause inflammation and ulcers in the GI tract. The most common disorders are ulcerative colitis and Crohn's disease.

insoluble A type of fiber that doesn't dissolve in water. Insoluble fiber is found in whole-grain products and vegetables.

intestinal flora The name for the bacteria, yeasts, and fungi that normally grow in the intestinal tract.

intestinal mucosa (intestinal lining) The surface lining of the intestines where the process of absorption occurs.

intestinal transit time How fast or slow material moves through the intestines.

intestines The set of long, tube-shaped organs in the abdomen that include the small intestine and large intestine.

lactase An intestinal enzyme that is needed to digest lactose.

lactose A complex sugar found in milk and milk products (also the principal sugar found in these products). Lactose must be broken down into the simple sugars galactose and glucose to be absorbed.

lactose intolerance A common condition in which a person does not produce enough lactase to digest the lactose in milk or milk products. It is commonly associated with abdominal cramping and diarrhea after drinking milk or eating dairy products.

large intestine The part of the intestinal tract that extends from the ileum to the anus. The large intestine is divided into the appendix, cecum, colon (ascending, transverse, descending, and sigmoid), rectum, and anus. Also called the large bowel

laxatives Agents aimed at relieving constipation by regulating bowel function. Types of laxatives include fiber supplements, bulking agents, osmotics, stimulants, and emollients.

malabsorption A condition in which the intestine has a less that normal ability to digest or absorb foodstuffs, which reduces the nutrients a person receives. Unabsorbed food may cause diarrhea and gas.

microorganism An extremely small organism that is not visible to the naked eye.

motility The movement of food through the digestive tract.

mucus A clear, sticky discharge.

neuron Nerve cells that carry messages through the network of nerves through the body.

neurotransmitters A chemical such as serotonin and norepinephrine that is made by nerve cells and used to communicate with other cells

nocturnal pain Pain that occurs during the night.

noninvasive A term used to describe procedures that do not require any injection into or surgical penetration of the body.

norepinephrine A chemical transmitting across synapses between neurons.

obstruction Blockage or clogging of a vessel, duct, etc., that prevents liquids or solids from flowing through the area and results in a buildup of pressure above the obstruction.

occult bleeding (hidden bleeding) Bleeding that is not visible on gross inspection.

parasites Tiny organisms that live inside a larger organism.

peristalsis The rippling motion of muscles in the GI tract, characterized by the alternate contraction and relaxation of the muscles that propel the contents onward.

pituitary gland A pea-sized endocrine gland located at the base of the brain that regulates and controls secretion of hormones from other endocrine glands, which in turn regulate many body processes such as growth, metabolism, fertility, and the conversion of food into energy.

placebo A "dummy" treatment that is made to look, taste, or feel as similar as possible to the "real" treatment in order to give a clear picture of what the true effects of the "real" treatment actually are.

placebo effect The benefits, or the unpleasant symptoms, which occur as a result of undergoing a "dummy" treatment that lacks the active ingrediant of the real treatment.

platelets Particles that circulate in the blood that are able to stop bleeding by forming blood clots or scabs.

Platelets circulate in a normal state until injury occurs; they are then activated through a series of molecular events initiated by the injury.

polyps Any mass of tissue that protrudes from the mucous lining of an organ such as the intestine.

postprandial pain Abdominal pain occurring shortly after eating a meal.

progesterone A female reproductive hormone made by the ovaries that prepares the uterus for egg implantation and prevents further ovulation during pregnancy.

prostaglandins A group of potent hormonelike substances that are produced in various tissues. Prostaglandins show pressure activity, mediate inflammation, and contract smooth muscles within the body.

receptor A molecule inside or on the surface of a cell that binds to a specific substance and causes a specific physiologic effect in the cell.

rectum The extreme lower end of the large intestine leading to the anus.

rheumatoid arthritis A chronic autoimmune disease that causes pain, swelling, stiffness, and loss of function in the joints.

Rome III Diagnostic Criteria A set of guidelines developed by a group of international GI experts to help diagnose irritable bowel syndrome and other functional GI disorders based on their specific symptoms.

serotonin A neurotransmitter that is densely concentrated in the gut and helps regulate mood, sleep, GI activity, pain perception, and appetite.

sigmoidoscope A rigid or flexible endoscope used to look into the anus, rectum, and sigmoid colon (the lower third of the colon). It may also have a tool to remove tissue to be checked under a microscope for signs of disease.

sigmoidoscopy A diagnostic procedure used to find a physical cause of diarrhea, abdominal pain, or constipation. Used to look for early signs of cancer in the descending colon and rectum.

small bowel follow-through A diagnostic procedure in which x-rays are taken of the small intestine as the barium liquid passes through it.

small intestine The largest part of the digestive tube that connects the stomach to the large intestine. The small intestine is divided into the duodenum, jejunum, and the ileum and is the site where most of the digestion and food absorption occurs.

soluble fiber A fiber that dissolves in water. Soluble fiber is found in beans, fruit, and oat products.

spasms Muscle movements such as those in the colon that are believed to cause pain, cramps, and diarrhea.

sphincter A ringlike band of muscles that constricts a passage or closes a natural body opening.

stomach The organ between the esophagus and the small intestine. The stomach is where acid is produced and digestion of protein begins.

stool The solid wastes that pass through the rectum during bowel movements. Stool is undigested foods, bacteria, mucus, and dead cells. Also called feces.

stress Reaction of the brain and body to adjust to the pressures or demands of one's environment. Stress is experienced by everyone and can be expressed in behavior, emotional, and or physical changes.

synapse The small gap between neurons where impulses cross over to communicate messages through the nervous system.

syndrome A group of symptoms that points to a specific medical diagnosis.

testosterone A male reproductive hormone that is produced in the testicles and is responsible for the development of secondary male sexual characteristics.

thyroid stimulating hormone (TSH) A hormone produced by the pituitary gland that stimulates the thyroid to produce thyroid hormones T3 and T4. When a thyroid disorder is suspected clinically, a TSH level is obtained as an initial test.

ulcer An open sore on the skin surface or on a mucous surface such as the lining of the stomach.

ulcerative colitis A serious disease that causes ulcers and inflammation in the inner lining of the colon and rectum. *See also* **inflammatory bowel disease (IBD)**.

ultrasound (ultrasonic imaging, echoscanning, ultrasonography) A diagnostic test in which sound pulses are sent into the body. The returning echoes are collected and a picture is produced from them. Ultrasound uses the same technology as sonar.

upper GI series *See* **barium meal.**

urinary retention Difficulty passing urine.

white blood cell Refers to a blood cell that does not contain hemoglobin. White blood cells are made by bone marrow and help the body fight infection and other diseases.

Your Daily IBS Diary

IBS SEVERITY SCALE

0	1	2	3	4	5	6	7	8
NONE		MILD		MODERATE		STRONG		SEVERE

For each day, rate how much of a problem each symptom is using the 0-8 severity scale.

Day	Pain or Discomfort	Diarrhea	Constipation	Sudden Urges	Bloating	Medication (type/amount)
Week #						
Mon						
Tue						
Wed						
Thu						
Fri						
Sat						
Sun						
Week #						
Mon						
Tue						
Wed						
Thu						
Fri						
Sat						
Sun						
Week #						
Mon						
Tue						
Wed						
Thu						
Fri						
Sat						
Sun						

Daily Stress Worksheet

Date	What was the event?	What thoughts or images crossed your mind during and after the event?	What were your physical sensations while it was happening?	What were your feelings while it was happening?	What did you do to handle your feelings, thoughts, or bodily sensations?

Relaxation Training Worksheet

	0	10	20	30	40	50	60	70	80	90	100
	None			**Mild**		**Moderate**			**Strong**		**Extreme**

Rate your relaxation and concentration using the above scale each time you practice.
In the last column, jot down anything that happens while you practiced.

Date	Practice Session	Relaxation at end of practice session	Concentration during practice session	Comments
	First			
	Second			
	First			
	Second			
	First			
	Second			
	First			
	Second			
	First			
	Second			
	First			
	Second			
	First			
	Second			
	First			
	Second			
	First			
	Second			
	First			
	Second			
	First			
	Second			
	First			
	Second			
	First			
	Second			

Daily Thought Worksheet

	0 10 20 30	40 50 60 70 80 90 100	
	NO CHANCE	**DON'T KNOW**	**DEFINITE CHANCE**

What was the event or situation? (1)	Specific worry or negative thoughts? (2)	Initial odds? (3)	What is the evidence? How do I know for sure? Consider alternatives? (4)	Realistic odds? (5)

Decatastrophizing Worksheet

What was the situation or event?	Thoughts during the event?	Questions to ask yourself •Is situation time limited? •Is it manageable? •Can I let go? Do I have a choice? •How useful is the thought? •Is it worth developing stomach problems over?	Physical sensations after asking yourself questions?	Feelings after asking yourself questions?	What did you do?

Thought-Tracking Worksheet

Trigger Situation	Initial Worry/Thought	Type of Thinking Error		Questions to Ask Yourself ·Evidence (how do you know for sure)? ·Alternative viewpoint? ·Usefulness of belief? ·Can I shift perspective?	Did the expected negative event occur?
		Jumping to Conclusions	Blowing Out of Proportion		YES NO

Problem-Solving Worksheet

Key Questions to Ask Yourself	Problem
What is the problem? Be specific, clear, and concrete •What is bothering me? •Why is it a problem?	
How much control do I really have over this situation? •Am I taking on too much responsiblity for things I can't control? •Am I ignoring aspects of the problem that are under my control? •Is the goal under the scope of what I can do?	
What can I do? Be specific, clear, and concrete •Write down all the possible options (even if they seem silly or impossible). •No criticism or judging •Think quality not quality •Match the option to type of problem (controllable vs. uncontrollable)	
Think it over •What could happen with each option? (Consider the type of problem, time required, costs involved, effects on me personally, effects on others.)	
Make a decision •Pick a solution that's best for me (consider the consequences). •Don't wait for perfect solution—pick one that's "good enough."	
Now do it •Figure out what you need to carry out a solution and do it	
How did it go? •Am I satisfied? •If not, what else could I do?	

Challenging Core Beliefs Worksheet

Situation	Thoughts	What would it say about me if thoughts were true?	Type of Core Belief •Perfectionism •Illusion of control •Expecting approval	Alternative Thought •Reversing positions •Reframing •Usefulness of thought

Food Diary

Name _____

Day _____

Food and Amount	Time	Symptoms	Severity of Symptoms 1 2 3 4 5 Low High	Time	Treatment or Medication
Breakfast					
_____	____	_____	_____	____	_____
_____	____	_____	_____	____	_____
_____	____	_____	_____	____	_____
Mid-morning Snack					
_____	____	_____	_____	____	_____
_____	____	_____	_____	____	_____
_____	____	_____	_____	____	_____
Lunch					
_____	____	_____	_____	____	_____
_____	____	_____	_____	____	_____
_____	____	_____	_____	____	_____
Mid-afternoon Snack					
_____	____	_____	_____	____	_____
_____	____	_____	_____	____	_____
_____	____	_____	_____	____	_____
Dinner					
_____	____	_____	_____	____	_____
_____	____	_____	_____	____	_____
_____	____	_____	_____	____	_____
Evening Snack					
_____	____	_____	_____	____	_____
_____	____	_____	_____	____	_____

PATIENT RESOURCES

Patient Advocacy Organizations

International Foundation for Functional GI Disorders
P. O. Box 170864, Milwaukee, WI 53217, Phone: 888-964-2001
www.iffgd.org Email: iffgd@iffgd.org.
Offers a wealth of trustworthy and helpful information about IBS. They publish articles contributed by an international group of medical experts and offer an informative quarterly magazine. Calls and questions are welcome on their toll-free phone number or via email.

IBS Network
Unit 5, 53 Mowbray Street, Sheffield, S3 8EN, Phone: 0114 272 32 53
Email: info@ibsnetwork.org.uk
www.ibsnetwork.org.uk/portal/Home/tabid/36/Default.aspx
This UK-based organization provides information, support, and advice for IBS patients and their families.

Irritable Bowel Syndrome Self-Help Group
P.O. Box 94074, Toronto, Ontario, Canada M4N 3R1
Phone: 416-932-3311. www.ibsgroup.org
Works to provide social networking and information for individuals with IBS and other functional GI disorders. The website provides access to bulletin and chat boards, blogs, news, a book list and store, medication listing, clinical trial listings, brochures, and information.

Government, Educational, and Professional Organizations

American College of Gastroenterology
P.O. Box 342260, Bethesda, MD 20827-2260, Phone: 301-263-9000
www.acg.gi.org/patients/ibsrelief/
Provides patient resources that span the broad range of digestive diseases and conditions including IBS. Their website includes chapters from a digestive health "Web Book" written by experts. These chapters provide an in-depth review for patients and their families, including information about diagnosis and the latest treatment options.

American Gastroenterological Association
4930 Del Ray Avenue, Bethesda, MD 20814
Phone: 301-654-2055. www.gastro.org
The AGA's website includes a "Patient Center" where patients can download information about various disorders of the digestive system.

American Society of Colon and Rectal Surgeons
85 West Algonquin Road, Suite 50, Arlington Heights, IL 60005
Phone: 847-290-9184. www.fascrs.org
The organization's website includes educational materials and informational brochures about common GI diseases. http://fascrs.org/displaycommon.cfm?an=2

MedlinePlus
www.nlm.nih.gov/medlineplus/irritablebowelsyndrome.html
Links to a variety of information from the government and medical societies on
diagnosis, symptoms, treatment, clinical trials, nutrition, disease management, and
occurrence in women and children.

National Digestive Diseases Information Clearinghouse
National Institutes of Health, 2 Information Way, Bethesda, MD 20892
Phone: 800-891-5389. www.niddk.nih.gov/health/digest/nddic.htm
An information dissemination service of the National Institute of Diabetes and
Digestive and Kidney Diseases. Established to increase knowledge and understanding
about digestive diseases among people with these conditions and their families, health-
care professionals, and the general public, NDDIC works closely with representatives
from federal agencies, voluntary organizations on the national level, and professional
groups to identify and respond to informational needs about digestive diseases.

UCLA Center for Neurovisceral Sciences & Women's Health
GLAVAHS, Building 115/CURE, Room 222A, 11301 Wilshire Boulevard,
Los Angeles, California 90073
Phone: 310-312-9276. www.ibs.med.ucla.edu/
Academic program that studies how the brain, stress, and emotions impact the
development of functional GI disorders like IBS and other related medical problems.
Its website includes informative resources for individuals interested in IBS and
coexisting medical problems.

University at Buffalo (SUNY) Behavioral Medicine Clinic
ECMC, 462 Grider Street, Buffalo, NY 14215
Phone: 716 898 6254 or -5671. www.wings.buffalo.edu/research/ibs/
A nationally known clinical-research facility devoted to research, education, and
treatment of painful medical disorders such as IBS. The clinic's primary academic
mission is to study the causes, underlying mechanisms, and treatments for IBS, and
to provide education and science-based resources for patients, their families, and
health-care professionals.

University of North Carolina Center for Functional GI & Motility Disorders
CB #7080, Bioinformatics Building, Chapel Hill, NC 27599-7080
Phone: 919-966-0144. www.med.unc.edu/medicine/fgidc/welcome.htm
Devoted to the study and treatment of functional GI disorders. One of its goals is
to produce helpful, up-to-date information for patients and the public through
seminars and workshops as well as printed materials, videos, and the Internet.

UpToDate
http://patients.uptodate.com/topic.asp?file=digestiv/8576
Online patient and professional information on medical topics including irritable bowel
syndrome.

www.nutrition.gov
Created by the National Agricultural Library, U.S. Department of Agriculture, this
website provides easy access to some of the best food and nutrition information on

the web. Users can find practical, current information on healthy eating, dietary supplements, and other lifestyle issues important to IBS patients.

NEWSLETTERS

Harvard Medical School publishes a number of quality monthly newsletters and special reports that frequently cover topics relevant to IBS patients. These newsletters include: *Harvard Health Letter, Harvard Women's Health Watch, Harvard Men's Health Watch.*

Tufts Health and Nutrition Letter is a publication from Tufts University, one of the most well respected schools of nutrition in the US. Provides readers with honest, reliable, scientifically authoritative health and nutrition advice and information.

UC Berkeley Wellness Letter provides accurate, current, and easy-to-understand information about the latest research in nutrition, health, and medicine. It examines the accuracy of fad diets and other anecdote-based regimens.

BOOKS

Conquering Irritable Bowel Syndrome: A Guide to Liberating Those Suffering with Chronic Stomach or Bowel Problems. Nicholas J. Talley, M.D., Ph.D. (B. C. Decker Inc., 2005)
Dr. Talley, Chair of Internal Medicine at the Mayo Clinic (Jacksonville, Florida) is a leading authority on IBS. The book provides information about the nature, symptoms, types and causes of IBS, diagnostic tests and medical options available to IBS patients.

Making Sense of IBS: A Physician Answers Your Questions about Irritable Bowel Syndrome. Brian E. Lacy, M.D., Ph.D. (Johns Hopkins University Press, 2006)
Dr. Lacy, a gastroenterologist at Dartmouth Medical School, has extensive clinical and research experience in the field of functional GI disorders. His book addresses many common questions patients have about IBS, including how IBS develops, how it is diagnosed, how symptoms are affected by stress, and the value of currently available treatments.

Rome III. The functional gastrointestinal disorders: Diagnosis, pathophysiology and treatment: A multinational consensus. (Degnon Associates, 2006.)
Email: romefoundation@degnon.org. Website: www.romecriteria.org
A valuable sourcebook of information on the epidemiology, pathophysiology, diagnosis, and treatment of irritable bowel syndrome and other functional GI disorders. Rome III is a comprehensive, authoritative guide to original source materials used in writing this book.

PODCASTS

http://www.ibstales.com/podcasts.htm
This podcast provides an autobiographical narrative of one person's life dealing with IBS.

SELECTED REFERENCES

Andresen, V., & Camilleri, M. (2006). Irritable bowel syndrome: recent and novel therapeutic approaches. Drugs, 66(8), 1073-1088.

Camilleri, M., Bueno, L., de Ponti, F., Fioramonti, J., Lydiard, R. B., & Tack, J. (2006). Pharmacological and pharmacokinetic aspects of functional gastrointestinal disorders. Gastroenterology, 130(5), 1421-1434.

Camilleri, M., & Spiller, R. C. (Eds.). (2002). Irritable bowel syndrome: Diagnosis and treatment. London: W. B. Sanders.

Cash, B. D., & Chey, W. D. (2005). Diagnosis of irritable bowel syndrome. Gastroenterol Clin North Am, 34(2), 205-220, vi.

Cheng, C., Hui, W., & Lam, S. (2000). Perceptual style and behavioral pattern of individuals with functional gastrointestinal disorders. Health Psychol, 19(2), 146-154.

Coates, M. D., Mahoney, C. R., Linden, D. R., Sampson, J. E., Chen, J., Blaszyk, H., et al. (2004). Molecular defects in mucosal serotonin content and decreased serotonin reuptake transporter in ulcerative colitis and irritable bowel syndrome. Gastroenterology, 126(7), 1657-1664.

Drossman, D. A., Corazziari, E., Talley, N. J., Thompson, W. G., & Whitehead, W. (2006). Rome III. The functional gastrointestinal disorders: Diagnosis, pathophysiology and treatment: A multinational consensus, (2 ed. ed.). McLean, VA:: Degnon Associates.

Gershon, M. D. (1998). The Second Brain. New York: HarperCollins.

International Foundation for Functional Gastrointestinal Disorders. (2002). IBS in the real world. Milwaukee, WI: IFFGD.

Lackner, J. M., Jaccard, J., Krasner, S. S., Katz, L. A., Gudleski, G. D., & Blanchard, E. B. (2007). How does cognitive behavior therapy for IBS work?: A mediational analysis of a randomized clinical trial. Gastroenterology, 133, 2, xxx-xxx.

Lackner, J. M., Lou Coad, M., Mertz, H. R., Wack, D. S., Katz, L. A., Krasner, S. S., et al. (2006). Cognitive therapy for irritable bowel syndrome is associated with reduced limbic activity, GI symptoms, and anxiety. Behav Res Ther, 44(5), 621-638.

Lacy, B. E. (2006). Making Sense of IBS: A Physician Answers Your Questions about Irritable Bowel Syndrome. Baltimore, MD,: A Johns Hopkins Press Health Book. Medicine Consumer Health.

Lazarus, R. S., & Folkman, S. (1984). Stress, appraisal, and coping. New York: Springer.

Lin, H. C. (2004). Small intestinal bacterial overgrowth: a framework for understanding irritable bowel syndrome. JAMA, 292(7), 852-858.

Maxwell, P. R., Mendall, M. A., & Kumar, D. (1997). Irritable bowel syndrome.

Lancet, 350(9092), 1691-1695.

Mayer, E. A., Naliboff, B. D., Chang, L., & Coutinho, S. V. (2001). V. Stress and irritable bowel syndrome. *Am J Physiol Gastrointest Liver Physiol, 280*(4), G519-524.

Mayer, E. A., Naliboff, B. D., & Craig, A. D. (2006). Neuroimaging of the brain-gut axis: from basic understanding to treatment of functional GI disorders. *Gastroenterology, 131*(6), 1925-1942.

McEwan, B., & Lasley, E. N. (2002). *The End of Stress As We Know It.* Washington, D. C.: Jospeh Henry Press.

Mertz, H. R. (2003). Irritable bowel syndrome. *N Engl J Med, 349*(22), 2136-2146.

Muller-Lissner, S. A., Kamm, M. A., Scarpignato, C., & Wald, A. (2005). Myths and misconceptions about chronic constipation. *Am J Gastroenterol, 100*(1), 232-242.

NIH Technology Assessment Panel on Integration of Behavioral and Relaxation Approaches into the Treatment of Chronic Pain and Insomnia. (1996). Integration of behavioral and relaxation approaches into the treatment of chronic pain and insomnia. *JAMA, 276*(4), 313-318.

Park, M. I., & Camilleri, M. (2006). Is there a role of food allergy in irritable bowel syndrome and functional dyspepsia? A systematic review. *Neurogastroenterol Motil, 18*(8), 595-607.

Quartero, A. O., Meineche-Schmidt, V., Muris, J., Rubin, G., & de Wit, N. (2005). Bulking agents, antispasmodic and antidepressant medication for the treatment of irritable bowel syndrome. *Cochrane Database Syst Rev*(2), CD003460.

Raphael, K. G. (2005). Childhood abuse and pain in adulthood: more than a modest relationship? *Clin J Pain, 21*(5), 371-373.

Schoenfeld, P. (2005). Bacterial overgrowth & IBS: Too soon to tell. *AGA Perspectives.*

Spiller, R. C. (2007). Role of infection in irritable bowel syndrome. *J Gastroenterol, 42 Suppl 17*, 41-47.

Tack, J., Broekaert, D., Fischler, B., Oudenhove, L. V., Gevers, A. M., & Janssens, J. (2006). A controlled crossover study of the selective serotonin reuptake inhibitor citalopram in irritable bowel syndrome. *Gut, 55*(8), 1095-1103.

Talley, N. (2006). *Conquering Irritable Bowel Syndrome.* Hamilton, ON,: B. C. Decker.